Wakefield Press

Default Depression

Anthony Smith, former board member of Suicide Prevention Australia, is at the forefront of a movement that aims to change the way we consider mental health and suicide prevention. He is co-author of papers and reports promoting the Situational Approach, a concept that offers a fresh way of considering mental health by taking situational factors (such as economic and social disadvantage, and workplace stress) into account when diagnosing and treating depression and anxiety disorders.

For more than two decades Anthony has worked across Australia with networks such as primary health, the life insurance industry, men's sheds and human resources, and at the community level in suicide prevention and research, built on collaborative work with a regional coroner's office.

Default Depression

How we now interpret human distress
as mental illness

Anthony Smith

Wakefield
Press

Wakefield Press
16 Rose Street
Mile End
South Australia 5031
www.wakefieldpress.com.au

First published 2023

Cover designed by Stacey Zass
Edited by Julia Beaven, Wakefield Press
Typeset by Michael Deves, Wakefield Press

ISBN 978 1 92304 200 1

A catalogue record for this
book is available from the
National Library of Australia

Wakefield Press thanks
Coriole Vineyards for
continued support

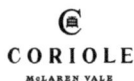

Contents

Preface

We now systematically interpret distress and common human behaviours and experience as symptomatic of clinical mental disorder. This is Default Depression. We do this on a large scale, and we do it through formalised policy and practice in every sector of our community. We direct distressed people into the restrictive pathway of a formal medical diagnosis – typically clinical depression, Default Depression – and then treat them with potentially harmful antidepressant drugs. In doing so, we largely disregard the causes of people's distress, the evidence challenging key aspects of the discrete category of clinical depression and the harms caused by antidepressant drugs.

The rise of 'depression' as a class of medical diagnosis and treatment has been a major social phenomenon and is now one of the most common diagnoses made by general practitioners (GPs) in most Western countries. The activity, messaging and system of beliefs around depression and mental illness have grown at such a rate and been applied so broadly that depression has become a standard formalised part of organisational policy throughout the breadth of sectors and settings in Western nations – far beyond the health and mental health sectors.

A key principle of this belief system is the presumption that the distress individuals experience is symptomatic of a mental disorder, including clinically diagnosable depression and anxiety. Further, mental disorder is presented as having a biological basis, thus treatable with drugs that can rectify a presumed chemical imbalance in the brain. This individualist approach disregards crucial social determinants of people's psychological and emotional wellbeing.

We seem to have lost sight of the fact that across the spectrum of human experience, people become distressed for a range of reasons – and that this is what it is to be human. Within the range of feelings of distress, people may experience a debilitating state of poor psychological or emotional wellbeing – they may feel *depressed*. This suffering is real, and these distressed individuals may need support, including possible medical or psychiatric support. Being distressed, however – even feeling depressed – does not and should not automatically presume a mental disorder. To diagnose this distress as a case of clinical depression and choose a restrictive medical pathway may well do more harm than good to many people. That we now routinely choose this approach to distress is Default Depression in action.

An integral component of Default Depression is the political and corporate activity that perpetuates a system of beliefs and practices built around contradictory evidence – to which the focus on depression is central. Key aspects of our current approach to mental health have even been described as 'ideological'.[1]

This increasingly entrenched pathway of identification, diagnosis and treatment of distress as a mental disorder has been a major factor in the escalating diagnoses of clinical depression and anxiety disorder, and the prescribing of antidepressants. And because this systemic approach to psychological and emotional distress, and the focus on depression, dominates the policy and practice of the suicide prevention sector, it also arguably contributes significantly to the challenges of effectively addressing the increasing numbers of suicide deaths. From 2006 to 2021 in Australia, there was an increase of around 35%, leading to more than 3000 suicide deaths in 2021.[2]

The pervasiveness of the illness paradigm in mental health has swamped suicide prevention efforts to the extent that suicide prevention has come to be seen as a logical extension of the mental health sector – as though distress exists on a continuum with suicide;

that suicidality is a clinically treatable mental health condition; and as though it is appropriate that the expertise and leadership required to address the tragedy of suicide deaths should be largely confined to mental health professionals or academics, generally with medical backgrounds. We need to broaden our view of the causality of suicide so that our prevention and response activity includes – but is not limited to – the health/mental health sector; and that leadership in the suicide prevention efforts should be expanded to include experts from outside this sector, who have a broader view of what is required to address these complex challenges.

An unquestioned focus on the interpretation of emotional and psychological distress as clinical mental disorder has also informed much of the current approach to workplace mental health. Depression has become a standard part of workplace health and safety, particularly via human resources; viewing worker distress as a clinical condition has become an automatic and unquestioned response – the *default* response, formalised in policy and practice – to complex workplace challenges. Meanwhile, the cause of the distress for the worker may be left unexamined. Common preventative practices include widespread workplace mental health training and formalised processes for identifying and 'treating' depression, with ongoing support for workers experiencing distress often being conditional on a formal diagnosis of a clinical mental disorder.[3] This institutionalisation of mental health in the workplace has had a profound impact on general medical practice, to the extent that mental health is now the main activity of general practice.[4]

The culture around workplace mental health has become an enormous, self-sustaining industry of considerable magnitude and influence, with training delivery, business planning and consultation processes – but the outcomes are questionable. There are increasing numbers of workers being directed to GPs for treatment of a mental disorder (commonly clinical depression), a highly problematic situation for people to find themselves in. Evidence shows the diagnosis of depression or any mental disorder severely restricts people's future employment opportunities;[5] the stigma of mental health is still a major burden,[6] and publicity campaigns about this issue appear to have had little effect. Workplace mental health policies have been developed to target individuals, and though this is partially driven by well-intentioned concern for people in distress, it fails to address the broader social context impacting on a worker's wellbeing, including, importantly, the conditions and dynamics of the workplace.

The scale of workplace mental health activity has also created an enormous cost burden to industry. There has been some attempt in recent years to investigate the impact of the current approach to mental illness on the workplace in Australia, particularly the financial sector, where the cost of income protection for workers' absence through diagnosis of mental disorder is now costing insurance companies over $500 million per year – and growing.[7] The enormous cost of escalating workplace mental health claims – contingent upon formal diagnoses of depression and other clinical mental 'disorders' – is causing such serious concerns that some leaders of the industry have gone on to publicly question the sustainability of the life insurance industry in its current form. A crucial dynamic in this context is the well-established partnership connection between the insurance industry and the superannuation industry as part of risk-management by insurance companies.[8] This business partnership (unique to Australia because of the magnitude of the superannuation sector) provides important support for workers. It is highly likely that the flow-on effect of the economic challenges to this sector through the escalating insurance claims for mental disorder will have a major detrimental impact on the super packages for workers throughout Australia, who may lose the insurance cover benefits, including income protection, that are currently offered as part of their superannuation package.[9]

The interpretation and treatment of human distress as clinical depression has taken place despite much concern, over many decades, about this approach. There have been volumes of published research challenging the very nature of the clinical categorisation itself. Along with this, there are serious concerns about the over-prescribing of antidepressants – the common treatment for both clinical depression *and* anxiety disorder – and the harm that this causes.[10] This is not to say there is no case at all for their use; rather, the concern is that antidepressant prescription is now at record levels, and too often issued as an automatic and unquestioned treatment to any number of behaviours and responses associated with stressful situations.[11] There were close to 40 million mental health-related prescriptions provided in Australia in 2017–2018.[12] Seventy per cent of these were antidepressant medications. Shockingly, these rates include over 100,000 children prescribed antidepressants, a marked increase in recent years.

There has been considerable concern about the opportunity cost; that the focus on depression and anxiety as a factor in compromised personal wellbeing ('mental ill-health') and suicide deaths has been at the expense of the development of strategies that may more effectively address these significant challenges.

This focus on mental health has led to a well-documented substantial increase in the diagnoses of clinical depression.[13] A recent survey shows that for the 2017/18 financial year, 20% of us (4.8 million Australians) had a mental or behavioural condition, an increase from 18% in 2014/15.[14]

There are a number of important concerns about this trend, and these include: inappropriate diagnoses,[15] challenges to general practice,[16] unhelpful screening tools,[17] the potential harms from prescription antidepressants, and the disregard for the social determinants of distress[18] – all of which compound the challenges of all these issues by rendering our current preventative efforts deficient and largely ineffective.[19]

Indeed, despite the many, many millions spent on the strategies and messages of the mental health/suicide prevention sector, there is very little debate about their merit or effectiveness. This is despite very clear data showing consistent rises in suicide death rates, diagnoses for depression, and prescribing of antidepressants. In fact, recent scathing evaluations of high-profile well-funded activities appear to have been completely ignored.[20]

In short, the mental health system is now heavily criticised from all sides.[21] It is sobering to know that in the most recent survey in 2011, the death rate due to intentional self-harm for those who accessed mental-health-related treatments was more than three times higher than that of the total Australian population.[22]

While there are a number of valuable books and theses that investigate some of the key themes around over diagnosing for mental disorders and the harms from antidepressants – many of which I have drawn upon in my research – this is the first major project to show how these trends have become institutionalised as policy and practice throughout our community, especially in workplace and organisational settings.

There are many who have been negatively impacted by the current approach to suicide prevention and mental health, but who have had limited alternative options for dealing with the distress in their lives because of the systemic nature of the current policies and practices. These include parents struggling to manage the challenges associated with the side effects of antidepressants on their children, or their children's withdrawal from the antidepressants; health professionals who have little in the way of referral options for patients other than further treatment within the health or mental health system; families and friends of people who have died by suicide, where there was little support available to help with the causes of their loved one's distress prior to their suicide death, other than medical treatment; and community activists, who have been hamstrung in their efforts to develop systems of support that target causal and situational factors for distress.

These voices and perspectives are largely unheard. Media covering mental health has a strong preference for high-profile leaders of the mental health/suicide prevention sector. These same figures also influence government and corporate policy, so media coverage and policy development are heavily influenced by people who endorse the current approach and disregard contrary expert opinions and evidence from lived experience. Enormous government, philanthropic and corporate funding (including from pharmaceutical companies) over the last several decades has gone into publicity campaigns promoting depression and mental health. A range of messages has been presented to the public as the appropriate approach (implying there is an authentic evidence-base) to tackle challenges around suicide deaths and mental health issues. Common themes include: people should visit their GP if they are 'down'; depression screening tools accurately identify mental disorders; men who are troubled should talk to someone about their feelings; workplace mental health training helps workers identify depression; depression is a 'condition' that can be identified and successfully treated with antidepressant drugs; antidepressant drugs are the appropriate treatment for depression; a person who has died by suicide must have had a mental illness; suicide death is an extreme form of self-harm; suicide prevention appropriately sits within the mental health system; the more people we train in suicide prevention the more effective we will be … The list goes on.

This messaging has been so effective that people from across the full spectrum of community and industry have taken the ideas on board as the acceptable and appropriate approach to the challenges of suicide prevention and mental health. Well-meaning practitioners and community activists in the mental health/suicide prevention sector have also accepted these messages, and so they, too, perpetuate the current approach. While there have been considerable challenges to many of the key concepts of the current approach, from both academia and the community, the criticisms and concerns appear to have been largely disregarded, and have had little influence on public messaging, and little bearing on the development of suicide prevention and mental health policy and practice. Concerns about the current approach are also not heard by academic researchers who are funded to research projects that align with the current approach where depression is a key topic. We read reports about how many people are depressed, but we hear very little about *why* they are depressed and how they are being treated once they are diagnosed.

Default Depression further contends that the general messages and strategies of the mental health/suicide prevention sector, rather than genuinely representing the breadth of available evidence and expert opinion, actually serve the substantial business interests of key organisations in the mental health/suicide prevention sector.

This book offers an alternative perspective to distress, and suggestions on how to develop more appropriate support. It seeks to counter myths about the Default Depression process and to expose vested interests in maintaining the current approach to mental health. That said, the book acknowledges that the medical system has a vital role in suicide prevention and supporting people in distress. There are a range of clinical mental illness conditions which, in severe cases, can have a seriously detrimental effect on the psychological and emotional wellbeing of people and can lead to self-harm and suicide. Examples of these all too real difficulties include some psychotic and schizophrenic experiences and severe depression with psychomotor retardation. It is vital for the welfare of people experiencing these difficulties to have an effective system for initial identification and engagement and, where appropriate, the provision of quality medical or psychiatric diagnosis and treatment.

The arguments and themes in this book are supported by a wealth of evidence and expert opinion from around the world that critique key aspects of our current approach to suicide prevention and mental health, and question some of the research methodologies and findings on which that approach is based. This evidence is complemented by critical analysis from other sources, including media articles and conversations with experts from a range of sectors including academia, human resources and primary health care, community-level activists, and from people with lived experience of suicide and self-harm and of the medicalised treatment of distress.

The dynamics and trends in this evidence mean that we urgently need wholesale change to how we support people in psychological and emotional distress, both within and beyond the mental health/ suicide prevention sector. We need a comprehensive national plan to address this challenge. While this is a huge undertaking needing strong support from government and business and community leaders, if we don't radically change our approach, the tragedy of increasing suicide deaths, the increasing harm from large-scale and often unnecessary use of antidepressant drugs, and the enormous social and economic cost of Default Depression will continue to increase. This book is intended to be a key resource for that process of change by contributing to a community voice that is calling for better, more effective support systems.

The Situational Approach

The Situational Approach provides a conceptual framework for considering suicide prevention and the challenges to providing appropriate support to people in psychological or emotional distress. This approach acknowledges the predominant association of situational distress with suicide, and is principally informed by and responds to risk factors of a broad spectrum of difficult human experiences across the life span. This approach is also mindful of – and, wherever possible, seeks to address – contextual, systemic, and sociocultural risk, as well as protective factors and determinants, such as family and relationship contexts, finances, health service availability and employment or employability – the real worlds of individuals' lived experience.

The Situational Approach to suicide prevention and mental health literacy therefore includes the complete spectrum of correlates of acute distress, from the broadest social factors to individual-level psychological and emotional factors. This approach to suicide prevention proposes that even in the most extreme cases of psychological or emotional difficulty, the social context of the distressed person must remain a priority in the consideration of developing appropriate support.

A note on terminology

Clarification around language and terminology is important to this topic and there are sections later in the book that deal with this in more detail. It is particularly important, however, that from the beginning there is clarity around the key term 'depression' as it is commonly understood, and the distinction from the term and category of 'clinical depression'.

People may experience a range of psychological or emotional difficulties related to a stressful situation or event, such as bereavement, a change in health status, relationship breakdown, financial or occupational difficulties. People may feel *down* or *troubled*, they may feel *depressed*. They may be grieving or having trouble sleeping ... Commonly, this distress is described as *depression;* as *being depressed.* The experience of psychological or emotional difficulty – the distress – may include feelings and sensations that significantly overlap with many of the symptoms taken to suggest clinical mental illness or disorder, such as clinical depression and anxiety disorder.

However, to limit the scope of understanding of this distress to that of a medical case of a clinical mental illness or disorder, and to diagnose people experiencing this kind of distress with a clinical disorder and treat them according to medical guidelines for that disorder, can compound people's difficulties. Even when the cause of this distress is seemingly inexplicable, it still doesn't necessarily represent what can be justifiably termed *illness* or *disorder.*

To feel *depressed* is a very different thing to having *clinical depression* – although common usage now often conflates the two and creates unhelpful ambiguity.

To minimise this ambiguity throughout the book, I maintain the distinction between the common usage of the term *depression* to describe a person who feels down or troubled, and *clinical depression,* which I use to refer to the formalised process of medical diagnosis for depression.

The confusion around these terms is further complicated by the ambiguous use of the term 'mental health'. There is a broad conflation between the general use of the term, which we generally understand to refer to a person's state of psychological or emotional wellbeing, and the more clinical medical use of the term, which infers an opposite, 'mental ill-health', and clinically diagnosable mental disorders. The confusion grows because the terms depression and mental health are often used interchangeably.

Where I can, I use the term 'psychological or emotional wellbeing' rather than 'mental health' as it applies to individuals.

Another frequently used term is 'suicide prevention': this is a broad term describing activities aimed at reducing the risk and prevalence of suicide, from prevention through to intervention and postvention (the support given to family and friends of someone who died by suicide). Suicide prevention and work in 'mental health' are often put together as part of the one sector of activity.

The term, the 'current approach' as used in this book, encompasses the overall culture of the mental health/suicide prevention sector and how we currently approach suicide prevention and mental health work through: program and campaign design; funding of research and 'preventative' projects; the policies we develop; and the people and organisations held up as experts.

Chapter 1

The limits of the current approach to suicide prevention

There is strong evidence showing that key aspects of the current approach to suicide prevention, particularly directing people in distress into the mental health system, may have tragic outcomes.[1] Key limitations of the current approach are explored in this chapter. Further limitations that stifle efforts to work toward more effective suicide prevention will be explored in more detail in the Situational Approach content in Chapter 9.

Current limitations include:

- *the unnecessary and potentially harmful medicalisation and pathological categorisation of human distress, and disregard for the situational and dimensional nature of human experience*
- *the conflation of mental illness and suicide*
- *significant neglect of primary and secondary prevention efforts in favour of crisis intervention, which leaves those most vulnerable to mental health difficulties and suicide to simply 'fall through the cracks'*
- *a failure to properly recognise and enlist the preventative potential of human service agencies and organisations outside the mental health field such as housing, re-employment support, legal and financial service support*
- *over-reliance on mental illness perspectives from the mental health sector in suicide prevention, and disregard for expertise relevant to a broader perspective on suicide and effective suicide prevention*

1

- *the increasing phenomenon of non-health and non-mental health organisations (influenced by mental health literacy messaging) directing clients to GPs rather than other more appropriate support services*
- *suicide prevention and mental health training programs that continue to present perspectives that have significant inherent problems and contradictions and have been shown to be ineffectual in suicide prevention.*[2]

Around the world there has been an increased focus and clearly stated community priorities aimed at elevating the profile of suicide prevention. The World Health Organization (WHO) has explicitly encouraged countries to place suicide prevention high on their agenda.[3] And the national governments of the US, Canada and the UK have recently published strong policies promoting suicide prevention and outlined considerable government support.[4]

In Australia there have been similar strong moves at both federal and state levels to increase suicide prevention and here, too, this has been supported by substantial increases in budgets. In 2019, the federal government invested $461 million into a Youth Mental Health and Suicide Prevention Plan as part of the 2019/2020 Budget.[5] The funding directed into suicide prevention activity in Australia has continued to grow for more than a decade.[6]

And yet, despite the increasing focus and budgets for mental health, if assessed by the key and surely most meaningful measure – numbers of suicide deaths per year – the current approach to suicide prevention in Australia is failing badly. Despite spending large amounts of government, corporate and philanthropic money there has been a disturbing, consistent upward trend in suicide deaths in Australia for almost the last two decades, with an alarming 31% increase between 2004 and 2017.[7] Suicide deaths now total around 3000 or more per annum,[8] about twice the number of fatalities from all motor vehicle accidents and homicides combined. During 2021, 3144 people died by suicide in Australia.

In 2016, the cost of suicide deaths in Australia was calculated at $1.6 billion, with the cost of youth suicide in 2014 estimated at $511 million a year.[9]

This trend is reflected around the globe, with the number of suicide deaths increasing by 6.7% globally between 1990 and 2016.[10] Suicide was the leading cause of potential years of life lost due to premature death in the Global Burden of Disease Study in the high-income Asia Pacific, and was among the top 10 leading causes of death in Eastern Europe, Central Europe, Western Europe, Central Asia, Australasia, Southern Latin America, and high-income North America. The suicide rates in US have increased 33% between 1999 and 2016.[11]

Even in some countries where the rates had been falling for the majority of the 21st century they have more recently begun rising again. In the UK, the suicide rate has recently risen by 10.9%, with the male and female suicide rates increasing by 11 and 10.2% respectively between 2017 and 2018.[12]

Many current suicide prevention initiatives (and associated 'mental illness' messaging) continue to strongly conflate mental illness with suicide, and offer little support to individuals experiencing suicidal ideation other than that based around medical treatment for a mental disorder. The authors of 'Suicide and mental disorders: A discourse of politics, power, and vested interests', a paper published in the *Death Studies* journal in 2017, state in their conclusion that 'the discourse on the relationship between mental disorders and suicide is permeated with ideology, politics, and power positioning suicide as a predominately medical/psychiatric issue'.[13]

Efforts to revitalise the current approach to suicide prevention with new evidence-based policies and strategies have generally been treated as peripheral, tempered to suit the current approach, or disregarded. The suicide prevention sector has become highly politicised, and powerful well-funded organisations work strategically to ensure their agenda dominates the business and activity of the sector, while alternative possibilities for the development of more effective suicide prevention activity are not given due consideration.[14]

There is an argument to say that in maintaining a focus on issues such as depression, while excluding key social determinants, these organisations have become a part of the problem.

Recent years have also seen increases in the profile and funding for the mental health/suicide prevention sector. That these trends correlate is no coincidence – they are driven by a set of interrelated dynamics that support and perpetuate a paradigm of deficiency and illness. These dynamics include marketing, policy development, program activity, media campaigns and funding of research, as well as the more recent development of the workplace as a major setting for identifying and encouraging medical treatment of depression.

A strong statement from the United Nations in 2017 corroborates this view:

> Regrettably, recent decades have been marked with excessive medicalization of mental health and the overuse of biomedical interventions, including in the treatment of depression and suicide prevention. The biased and selective use of research outcomes has negatively influenced mental health policies and services. Important stakeholders, including the general public, rights holders using mental health services, policymakers, medical students, and medical doctors have been misinformed. The use of psychotropic medications as the first line treatment for depression and other conditions is, quite simply, unsupported by the evidence. The excessive use of medications and other biomedical interventions, based on a reductive neurobiological paradigm, causes more harm than good, undermines the right to health, and must be abandoned.[15]

The workplace mental health context has contributed significantly to the substantial increases in diagnoses of clinical depression and anxiety disorder and the prescription of potentially harmful antidepressant drugs. And the leadership of the mental health/suicide prevention sector has been a major driver in the comprehensive cultural and institutional change across all industry sectors through workplace mental health. The mental health/suicide prevention sector is itself driven by a well-funded focus on depression, to the extent that funding for prevention efforts has been directed to depression-related activity, largely to the exclusion of developing potentially more effective prevention activity targeting evidence-based social correlates. The development of the current approach in a number of Western countries has been heavily influenced by business interests, including those of pharmaceutical companies and mental health training providers. This dynamic is explored in more detail in the recent book *Overprescribing Madness: What's driving Australia's mental illness epidemic?* by Martin Whitely,[16] and an award-winning PhD thesis by Melissa Raven,[17] both addressed later in this book.

Calculating precisely how much money is spent (or wasted) addressing suicide prevention specifically is hard to quantify. What we do know is government budgets for mental health and suicide prevention in Australia now amount to hundreds of millions of dollars per year, an all-time high.[18]

Crucially, major players in the mental health/suicide prevention sector have substantial budgets amounting to tens of millions of dollars per year; Beyond Blue, for example, had annual revenue of $60 million in 2019 and $65 million in 2018, and Black Dog Institute had annual revenue of $28 million in 2018/2019.[19] Unfortunately, despite expressions of support for the idea of social determinants of health/ mental health from the federal government, much of the federal 2020 funding for research to improve mental health care and reduce suicide rates in Australia still goes toward activities that sit within the mental illness paradigm, such as drug research for drug treatment, or simplistic one-dimensional ideas such as 'encourage men to seek help' without a thorough critique of whether or not existing services are actually helpful to men.[20]

As a nation we should demand a thorough review process of all aspects of the mental health/suicide prevention sector, including an economic analysis of the social and economic outcomes return on the financial investment into this sector.

The limits of the biomedical approach

The current approach to suicide prevention in Australia and much of the rest of the world is dominated by the biomedical approach. This generally refers to an approach in which health concerns are held to reside within the domain of the individual; that they are biological in nature and are treatable by medical means such as surgery and/or drugs.

The biomedical approach interprets psychological distress as symptomatic of a disorder or illness of some kind requiring diagnosis and treatment. This individualised approach tends to ignore social, contextual or situational factors and influences, reinforcing the assumption of a disordered organism, and pathologising and medicalising common human experience. Thus, this paradigm corrals the bulk of psychological distress into the diagnostic category of affective disorders (also known as mood disorders), largely depression, with some anxiety disorders. All of these are commonly referred to as 'disorders' or 'illnesses'. Of these, depression in particular is often presented as being associated with suicide not as a possible correlate, but as a causal factor. The conflation of so-called 'mental illness' with suicide continues to be a prime reason for the failure of so many suicide prevention enterprises, because it diverts attention away from the pathways of most suicides, which are predominantly characterised by psychological distress, rather than 'mental illness'.

Concerns about the biomedical approach to suicide have been growing. In general, these critiques suggest that this approach lacks a sound basis of evidence, and at best it can be characterised as a pseudoscientific ideology.[21] Unfortunately, like many ideologies, the current approach has significant negative consequences for many individuals, communities and societies; and in the case of suicide, may be responsible for escalating rather than mitigating risk in vulnerable individuals.

It is pertinent to read what the United Nations has to say about this issue as recently as 2017:

The biomedical model regards neurobiological aspects and processes as the explanation for mental conditions and the basis for interventions. It was believed that biomedical explanations, such as 'chemical imbalance', would bring mental health closer to physical health and general medicine, gradually eliminating stigma. However, that has not happened and many of the concepts supporting the biomedical model in mental health have failed to be confirmed by further research. Diagnostic tools, such as the *International Classification of Diseases and the* Diagnostic and Statistical Manual of Mental Disorders, *continue to expand the parameters of individual diagnosis, often without a solid scientific basis. Critics warn that the overexpansion of diagnostic categories encroaches upon human experience in a way that could lead to a narrowing acceptance of human diversity.*[22]

The UN report explicitly states that 'the field of mental health continues to be over-medicalised and the reductionist biomedical model, with support from psychiatry and the pharmaceutical industry, dominates clinical practice, policy, research agendas, medical education and investment in mental health around the world'. Other researchers in the field of suicide prevention offer similar considerations:

we routinely speak about evidence-based practices, risk management, assessment and treatment, monitoring, expert interventions, and scientific approaches to the study and prevention of suicide. While none of these approaches are inherently wrong, they are all generally grounded in an expert, biomedical framework and thus tend to narrow the range of possibilities for thinking about and responding to suicide.[23]

The current approach is largely a treatment paradigm – it aims to identify and treat individuals and disregards important social determinants that impact on their psychological wellbeing. The UN explicitly calls for a shift away from this approach to one that prioritises policy at the population level and targets social determinants:

Interventions are needed that avoid medicalizing emotional pain and empower individuals in vulnerable situations. Prevention strategies should prioritize addressing health determinants and improving human living conditions over those that disempower individuals and perpetuate social exclusion and stigma by pathologizing diverse responses to adversity.[24]

Biomedical explanations of psychopathology can have a detrimental impact in clinical practice. Authors Lebowitz and Appelbaum, in a 2019 paper in the *Annual Review of Clinical Psychology*, describe some of these consequences:

[Biomedical explanations of psychopathology] may also reduce clinicians' empathy for patients and lead clinicians to appear less warm, potentially interfering with therapist-patient relationships; and they appear to affect treatment preferences, leading to increased confidence in pharmacotherapy and decreased confidence in psychotherapy. In some studies, they also appear to reduce people's confidence in their own ability to overcome their symptoms. All of these effects have stark and potentially worrying clinical implications.[25]

Some researchers argue that there is an over-emphasis on individual traits and psychological qualities, and insufficient examination of the ways in which history, contexts, policies, discourses, and structures contribute to vulnerability, hopelessness and distress.[26] Most suicide prevention practices continue to be based on theorising at the individual level, generating solutions that emphasise individual responsibility, self-monitoring and seeking expert assistance.

Disregard for the social determinants of distress

Over the last few decades, there has been a growing trend to consider the concept of the social determinants of health. The fundamental idea of the social determinants of health is that the quality of health cannot be considered without acknowledgement of the social context of the lives and living circumstances of all people. The World Health

Organization (WHO), which has been active in raising the profile of the social determinants of health for some time, provides the following definition:

> *The social determinants of health (SDH) are the conditions in which people are born, grow, work, live, and age, and the wider set of forces and systems shaping the conditions of daily life. These forces and systems include economic policies and systems, development agendas, social norms, social policies and political systems.*[27]

More recently this same thinking is being applied to mental health; that is, that the social and political context of individuals has a fundamental place in their psychological and emotional wellbeing.[28] The WHO has also worked to raise the profile of social determinants of mental health as well:

> *levels of mental distress among communities need to be understood less in terms of individual pathology and more as a response to relative deprivation and social injustice, which erode the emotional, spiritual and intellectual resources essential to psychological wellbeing.*[29]

Despite research and clear statements from the WHO and the UN showing the vital importance of social determinants in good psychological wellbeing, the history of suicide prevention, with its focus on individual mental health, has largely been to disregard the social determinants. The Australian Government Department of Veterans Affairs echoes this concern.[30] There has been an effort made to direct prevention toward a more public health orientation, and to consider the cumulative effect of multiple pathways toward a state of despair.[31] However, while these trends are encouraging, the paradigm of illness in mental health still influences much of the thinking of the mental health/suicide prevention sector. And despite recent literature and media releases suggesting an increased consideration of social determinants, much of the focus is still on depression, with media and academics continuing to push this line.[32] The paradigm of illness is so deeply entrenched, that even where there is the acknowledgement of the social context in wellbeing, the language of the disorder/treatment paradigm is still central to some of the key literature.

> *Underlying the concept of the social determinants of mental health is the importance of a population-based, public health approach in identifying and treating mental disorders.*[33]

Data collection still looks at individuals and their presumed mental disorder and largely disregards social determinants. The Australian Bureau of Statistics for example, in collecting information for Cause of Death, has survey questions that focus on mental disorder and disregard social factors such as unemployment, even though unemployment is acknowledged in the international literature to be a major factor in suicide deaths (see Appendix A).[34]

Accurate data from the National Coronial Information System shows that suicide deaths among adults who are not employed account for at least 55% of all suicide deaths of people of working age in Australia (see Appendix B). There are even higher rates – 68.2% – of suicide deaths among women of working age who are not employed.[35] International research shows that unemployment is a significant factor in suicides in many Western countries and that providing appropriate support for those who are not employed can impact on suicide rates.[36] However, despite the easily accessible evidence showing that the majority of suicide deaths in Australia are people who are not employed, and the strong evidence for addressing unemployment as an effective means of addressing suicide deaths, there is nothing of any substance or appropriate scale done in Australia to address suicide deaths among those who are not employed – and calls over time to redress this have been simply disregarded.

The regular disregard of the social determinants of suicide in favour of the current approach has been raised as an ethical issue; that value judgements made in research and political decision-making that exclude evidence for the social determinants of suicide not only produce ineffective suicide prevention efforts but also constitute a major ethical dilemma for public health.[37] The example of unemployment as a factor in suicide deaths is a case in point; we have clear evidence of the lack of employment being a major factor in suicide deaths – and yet very little is done to address this.

The concept of the social determinants of mental health offers a genuine opportunity to address the substantial barriers to developing effective work in the mental health/suicide prevention sector. However, we need to ensure that debate around social determinants of mental health is not merely tokenistic. Key organisations in the mental health/ suicide prevention sector have been acknowledging social factors for the best part of two decades without really modifying their core activities, which remain focused on mental health.

Conceptual approaches to the range of suicide prevention activity

Suicide prevention activity operates across a spectrum from broader population-based preventative activity (to minimise people's increased risk of suicide in the first place) through to direct intervention with individuals already identified as having an elevated risk of suicide. The similarities of common conceptual approaches are illustrated in the figure below.

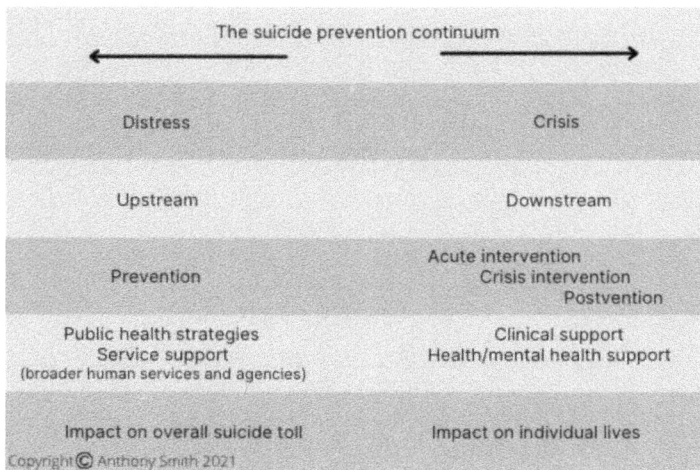

The suicide prevention continuum	
Distress	Crisis
Upstream	Downstream
Prevention	Acute intervention Crisis intervention Postvention
Public health strategies Service support (broader human services and agencies)	Clinical support Health/mental health support
Impact on overall suicide toll	Impact on individual lives

Copyright © Anthony Smith 2021

Figure 1. The suicide prevention spectrum

The predominance of acute intervention

One of the important limits of concern is that there is too great a focus on the acute – or crisis – end of the suicide prevention spectrum. The current approach is characterised by a:

> *predominance of tertiary suicide prevention services aimed at working with people who have already attempted suicide, have a high intensity mental health difficulty, or those bereaved by suicide (termed postvention support). Such services are certainly important, but will contribute little to diminishing the national suicide death toll.*[38]

Activity at the acute intervention stage is sometimes known as the 'downstream' end of the suicide prevention work. This work is certainly important, but on its own will contribute little to diminishing the national suicide death toll and is too often promoted and supported at the expense of more upstream prevention activity. The WHO reports that more than half of the interventions studied in a systematic review of suicide preventive interventions across the 'whole spectrum of suicide prevention efforts' fell into the domain of treatment and maintenance (acute intervention), rather than prevention.[39]

In recent years, there has been publicity and promotion of the idea of moving to a more 'upstream' focus for suicide prevention. This will need acknowledgment of the central role that socioeconomic factors play in mental health. MacIntyre et al argue that:

> *advancing 'upstream' approaches to population mental health requires an interdisciplinary research vision that supports greater understanding of the role of socioeconomic factors. It also demands collective cross-sectoral action through changes in social and economic policy, as well as economic frameworks that move beyond an exclusive focus on economic growth to embrace collective and societal wellbeing.*[40]

Recent acknowledgement of the importance of the social determinants influencing suicide offers hope that the necessary change in the suicide prevention sector is possible. However the well-established organisations presiding over the current approach (those favoured by government funding and decision-making) have proven to be resistant and obstructive to change. Addressing this inappropriate disbursement of funding and favour is a major challenge to improving the effectiveness of this sector. Despite the language of social determinants and upstream prevention, activity at the community level is still constrained by a focus on the depression of individuals, with messaging and programs around building individual resilience and encouraging individuals to talk about their mental health.

In Australia, we have some very good follow-up support (also known as 'postvention') for those affected by suicide but, like crisis-level intervention, this is often confused or conflated with prevention. And while some postvention and crisis-level interventions have some preventative benefit (for example, for family and friends of suicides who may be at an increased risk themselves), even the best quality follow-up support can never impact on the overall toll of suicide deaths, which requires commitment to effective upstream prevention. This definitional confusion serves to perpetuate some of the key dynamics of the current approach, and the unfortunate upward trend in suicide deaths continues. And not only is the current approach *not* helping reduce the toll of suicide deaths, but:

> *Suicide rates are either increasing or continuing unabated in many parts of the world. It is clear that narrow, risk factor-based approaches to suicide prevention are limited. We argue that they over-emphasize individual traits and psychological qualities, and neglect to examine the ways that history, contexts, policies, discourses, and structures contribute to vulnerability, hopelessness, and distress.*[41]

The limits of suicide prevention research and the prevalence of misinformation

Current suicide prevention research has been heavily criticised.[42] In the first instance, the dominance of the biomedical approach heavily influences the type of research done and a focus on mental health in research, particularly depression, has been heavily favoured.

Associated limits to the current approach to research include concerns about the methodology and the disregard for social determinants of distress.[43]

The current approach to suicide prevention research perpetuates the organisational and business status and profile of the leadership and key organisations in the mental health/suicide prevention sector too. 'Cherry-picking' of evidence to support the agendas of this leadership is common practice; certain aspects of the overall available data are highlighted, while others are downplayed. We have seen how data from the National Coronial Information System clearly shows how the lack of employment is a factor in over 50% of deaths, yet this is rarely presented in the literature. Meanwhile, data relating to rates of mental disorder are commonly cited. Ambiguity, misinformation and distorted perspectives abound.

The predominance of published research favours the current illness paradigm to the general exclusion of a broader conceptual framework. Let's look at the multiple ways the current approach promulgates misinformation:

The limits of data collection

The fundamental design of key survey tools is often skewed toward mental disorder and away from social determinants. In Australia, the Australian Bureau of Statistics presents data on Cause of Death and Suicide under the heading of intentional self-harm.[44] However, the causes of death presented are very much limited to the presence of mental disorders. Largely disregarded are known significant factors and clearly identifiable adverse life events and social determinants such as unemployment (see Appendix A). Gathering, analysing and presenting data with integrity is vital for effective suicide prevention.

The prevalence of unsubstantiated information

The figure of '90% of all suicides are depression/mental illness/mental disorder' has been commonly sprouted to justify the mental illness narrative as a basic framework for suicide prevention. This figure is unsubstantiated but is based on what is called the psychological autopsy approach to gathering suicide data – Information about the deceased is gathered through interviewing key informants, generally acquaintances of the deceased. However, despite the discrediting of the psychological autopsy approach to gathering suicide data,[45] various forms of the '90%' figure are still commonly cited and published in peer-reviewed journals. Further, there is no effort made by the leadership of the suicide prevention sector to invalidate this unhelpful misinformation.

The ambiguous use of rates and numbers

The misuse of 'rates' and absolute 'numbers' is very common. Both rates and numbers of suicide deaths are important considerations for appropriate suicide prevention activity. However, each considered alone without reference to the other can give a distorted view of suicide deaths. Commonly in the current approach, rates and numbers are used selectively and can, and often do, give a limited or even distorted view of the phenomenon of suicide deaths.

A good example of this is the common comparisons that are made between metropolitan and regional/rural suicides. While there is a great deal of information available about the relatively higher *rates* of suicide in rural and remote areas of Australia, there is very little information about the suicide rates in metropolitan areas. This is unfortunate, because it underplays the absolute dominance of the toll of suicide deaths that occurs in clearly defined geographical areas with low socio-economic standings in the major cities in Australia.[46] The five cities of Sydney, Melbourne, Brisbane, Adelaide and Perth together make up over half (54.18%) of all suicide deaths in Australia. It is true that in general, the regional/rural rate for suicide deaths is higher than for metropolitan areas. However, this is a considerable generalisation. Rates of suicide deaths vary enormously if measured by local government areas for both rural and metropolitan areas. Some metropolitan areas have both higher rates, as well as considerably higher numbers of suicide deaths than the general rural rates and numbers.

The conflation of self-harm with suicide deaths

There is a heavily gendered nature to the broad spectrum of self-harm from intentionally non-fatal self-harm through to suicide deaths. The majority – about 75% – of suicide deaths in Australia are of adult men (2358 of 3144 total suicide deaths in 2021).[47] In contrast, the majority of non-fatal self-harm incidents involve women and girls.[48] Compared with males, a larger proportion of females make a non-fatal suicide attempt.[49] Failing to make this distinction, and to not meaningfully take the gendered nature of suicide into account, perpetuates the ineffectiveness of current suicide prevention activity.

The category of self-harm includes non-fatal attempted suicide. While intentional self-harm is a high suicide risk factor,[50] the great majority of those with a history of self-harm do not go on to die by suicide[51] and the best available evidence suggests that the majority of completed suicides are first-time attempts.[52]

Severe psychiatric disorders are a factor in relatively few suicide deaths

Extensive research from Queensland shows that many men who die by suicide have no psychiatric history or known mental disorder – less than half of all these men had a diagnosed psychiatric condition.[53] People with severe psychological and emotional challenges who have been diagnosed as having a clinical psychiatric disorder such as schizophrenia and psychotic experiences do have an elevated risk of suicide, however, the proportion of suicides attributable to people living with severe psychiatric disorders is not clear. Statistical data that presumes 'psychiatric disorder' used historically has been discredited.[54] And the majority of diagnosed 'disorders' in suicide cases are classified as mood disorders – mainly depression – rather than more severe psychiatric disorders.[55]

The limitations of mental health apps and websites

Another major concern is the increasing attention on developing and promoting mental health apps; this is happening now on a large scale despite published research expressing serious concerns about their shortcomings. These include the lack of oversight on the development of new mental health apps and the consequent ever-expanding range of new and easily accessible apps, including those that promote the medicalisation of normal mental states, and others designed without an evidence base and that present inaccurate information.[56] Research published in 2021 outlines concerns about a number of clinically relevant metrics including privacy/security, effectiveness, and engagement. A media piece about this research describes the mental health app marketplace as a 'mess'.[57] Despite all of this, developing of apps appears to be popular with the leadership of the current approach and attracts considerable funding for development – again to the exclusion of approaches potentially more effective.

Similarly, many mental health websites are unhelpful. A 2020 investigation into information about antidepressants on popular websites published in the *International Journal of Risk & Safety* found:

> *None of the websites met our predefined criteria. The information was generally inaccurate and unhelpful and has potential to lead to inappropriate use and overuse of antidepressants and reduce the likelihood that people will seek better options for depression like psychotherapy.*[58]

Chapter 2

Distress as clinical disorder: a history and critique of the clinical approach to depression and anxiety

At the heart of this book is the fundamental question about the validity of key aspects of the clinical category of 'depression'. People often experience a range of troubling feelings that result in professionals describing them as 'being depressed'. However clinical categorisation presumes that there is a distinct state of mind that can be formally diagnosed and treated as a medical condition. While very little of general practice was taken up with treating depression in the first half of the 20th century, this is no longer the case. In Australia, treating mental health concerns has now become the dominant activity of general practice, with depression being the mental-health-related problem that GPs most frequently manage.[1]

There has been a great deal of valuable material already published about this issue, some of which is summarised in this chapter.[2] But it is also my intention to illustrate the dynamics that have driven this issue beyond the medical sector to become a factor across the whole community as formalised workplace and organisational policy and practice, and that has further driven the escalating rates of diagnosis of clinical depression and the consequential prescribing of antidepressants.

In increasingly large numbers, people in distress present themselves to GPs. On an individual level, they are encouraged to do this by public health messaging if they 'have the symptoms of depression'; on an institutional level, workplaces and organisational policy now direct distressed workers to GPs. On an enormous scale across the globe, doctors interpret the behaviours and responses to distress as symptoms of clinical depression, regardless of the cause of the distress, and then commonly treat this with antidepressants drugs.

From an Australian perspective, it is instructive to look at a real example of how we diagnose individuals for clinical depression to determine our national rates of depression.

- depressed mood
- loss of interest in activities
- lack of energy or increased fatigue
- loss of confidence or self esteem
- feelings of self-reproach or excessive guilt
- thoughts of death or suicide, or suicide attempts
- diminished ability to concentrate, think or make decisions
- change in psychomotor activity; agitation or retardation
- sleep disturbance
- change in appetite

The survey collected information to differentiate between three different types of Depressive Episode, based on the number of symptoms the person experienced:

- Severe Depressive Episode – all of the first three symptoms from the above list and additional symptoms from the remainder of the list to give a total of at least eight.
- Moderate Depressive Episode – at least two of the first three symptoms from the above list and additional symptoms from the remainder of the list to give a total of at least six.
- Mild Depressive Episode – at least two of the first three symptoms from the above list and additional symptoms from the remainder of the list to give a total of at least four.

Figure 2. List of symptoms for a depressive episode, Australian Bureau of Statistics Survey of Mental Health and Wellbeing[3]

A simple examination of the list as described in this survey tool – essentially identical to many other depression screening tools currently in use – clearly shows that most of these so-called 'symptoms' are actually normal human responses to any number of common stressful situations in people's lives; it is stretching scientific integrity for these to be automatically considered symptomatic of medical pathology.[4] Consider the responses most people have to the loss of a loved one, the loss of employment, financial or legal difficulties, or the breakdown of a relationship ... the feelings experienced may well be similar or the same as any of the so-called 'symptoms' above.

Furthermore, there is likely to be a combination of some of these 'symptoms' in stressful situations. A person experiencing these listed symptoms may require a supportive, caring approach with a broad consideration of the circumstances that might have brought them to this state of distress. And yet what we commonly do is have the patient tick some of these behaviours and then, with a relatively small number of ticks, they are then diagnosed with clinical depression – a mental disorder. While this tick-box approach has been strongly criticised, it is now a commonly used process for diagnosing clinical depression and anxiety disorder.[5]

This process – the labelling of a person with a clinical mental illness such as clinical depression – has an enormous impact on their life. It is likely that it may never be erased from their personal details; it is set like concrete in their health/mental health record. They are probably going to have to acknowledge their mental disorder whenever applying for a job. And if the diagnosis has been applied to a child, it is likely the rest of their schooling will be impacted.

The widespread acceptance of depression as a legitimate and discrete clinically diagnosable disorder, along with the focus of depression in the mental health/suicide prevention sector, has enabled the institutionalisation of practices around depression – that is, the enculturation of Default Depression. However, there is very little open debate about this process despite strong published research that challenges fundamental aspects of this phenomenon.

Default Depression pervades right to the heart of our community:

- We run workplace mental health training to help workers 'identify symptoms of depression'.
- We hire 'mental health experts', and 'ambassadors' to speak at community meetings about depression.
- We direct large amounts of funding toward research about depression.
- We have policies at schools to deal with depression among schoolchildren.
- Many of our charity organisations have developed suicide prevention activities that are primarily focused on depression.
- We spend enormous amounts of funding on campaigns that publicise and promote depression.

The clinical category for depression is a construct that sits firmly within the biomedical paradigm. That this category suits the marketing of antidepressant drugs is no coincidence. There is very little biological or neurological basis for the clinical category of depression and considerable difference in opinion within the health science community about the validity of the science behind the construction of the category, with strong challenges to important theoretical issues such as research design, and practical considerations such as appropriate treatment.

This is not to say that the distress suffered by some of those who are diagnosed as having a clinical depression is not real or debilitating – rather that this distress is often not either a result of, or the cause of, a clinical mental disorder. To reduce the person's distress to a diagnosis of clinical depression, and offer treatment in the form of potentially harmful antidepressant drugs, may well compound the difficulties for the distressed person.

A key dynamic in the institutionalisation of depression and anxiety has been the elevation of the particular terms 'depression' and 'anxiety' from common usage to formalised clinical categories. While historically there had long been an awareness of a general malaise referred to in the literature as 'melancholia', and general symptoms of stress were sometimes acknowledged to contribute to personal psychological and emotional challenges, these were formerly not considered to constitute an official category of mental disorder.

From the 1950s on, however, medical industry interest in anxiety began to grow. Later, from the 1970s on, with the development of new drugs to treat depression and anxiety, and with the formalised defining of clinical depression, together with the huge marketing budgets of global pharmaceutical companies, depression overtook anxiety as a key part of general medical practice. The implications of which are explored later in the book.

The clinical category for depression has no biological basis

There is very little empirical support for a discrete and unambiguous biological or neurological condition of clinical depression and there is considerable criticism of psychiatric diagnostic labels. Dr Kate Allsopp, the lead researcher of a 2019 paper 'Psychiatric diagnosis scientifically meaningless' (published in the *Psychiatry Research* journal),[6] was quoted in a report about the research in *Science Daily* from the University of Liverpool:

Although diagnostic labels create the illusion of an explanation they are scientifically meaningless and can create stigma and prejudice.[7]

Her colleague and co-author, Professor Peter Kinderman, added:

This study provides yet more evidence that the biomedical diagnostic approach in psychiatry is not fit for purpose. Diagnoses frequently and uncritically reported as 'real illnesses' are in fact made on the basis of internally inconsistent, confused and contradictory patterns of largely arbitrary criteria. The diagnostic system wrongly assumes that all distress results from disorder, and relies heavily on subjective judgments about what is normal.

Instead of being founded on biology or neurology, clinical diagnosis for depression is generally based on a sum score of symptoms that are, in fact, common but imprecise descriptions of emotional or psychological experiences or states. Rather than being grounded in solid biological science, a key part of the process for establishing a formal clinical category in mental health is instead decided by an agreement of people representing the health sector, influential physicians who 'discern and describe disorders based on their clinical experience, with little attempt at precise definition or method-based research. The main method of forming diagnoses in modern psychiatric nosology [classification] has been by committee agreement, based sometimes on quite limited empirical research'.[8]

Because of the broad nature of the category of depression there are problems in classification, diagnosis and treatment. Consequently, patients are often treated with inappropriate drugs.[9] The very idea of depression generally, and specifically as a distinct medical category, is considered by some physicians and researchers to be inadequate as a basis for working with patients suffering psychological or emotional distress; a distress that has become interpreted as symptomatic of mental disorder.[10]

There are strongly opposing ideas around the fundamental questions of what depression is, what causes it, and how to treat it. Even some researchers who are advocates of the biomedical approach to psychological or emotion distress concur that there is no satisfactory agreement about what depression is or how to properly treat it. Depression has been described as 'a clinically and etiologically heterogeneous disorder'; that is to say, the definition is extremely broad.[11] For instance, the list of 'symptoms' outlined above by the Australian Bureau of Statistics, various combinations of which are taken to denote severe, moderate and mild depressive episodes, such as 'loss of interest in activities', is very broad, while the symptoms themselves are indefinite descriptions of commonly occurring human experience. A recent article published in *Frontiers of Psychiatry* highlights the ambiguity around symptoms and the challenge this creates for appropriate diagnosis:

We demonstrate substantial inconsistency in the inclusion and emphasis of symptoms assessed within disorders as well as considerable symptom overlap across disorder-specific tools. Within the same disorder, similarity scores across assessment tools ranged from 29% for assessment of bipolar disorder to a maximum of 58% for OCD. Furthermore, when looking across disorders, 60% of symptoms were assessed in at least half of all disorders illustrating the extensive overlap in symptom profiles between disorder-specific assessment tools. Biases in assessment toward emotional, cognitive, physical or behavioral symptoms were also observed, further adding to the heterogeneity across assessments.

The consequence of this inconsistent and heterogeneous assessment landscape is that it hinders clinical diagnosis and treatment and frustrates understanding of the social, environmental, and biological factors that contribute to mental health symptoms and disorders.[12]

Researchers have also found that some developers of clinical guidelines for depression have ignored key issues and evidence that challenges the validity of some clinical trials.[13] The efficacy of some drug treatment is questionable; first-line treatment for major depressive disorder often fails, with about half of patients with clinical depression requiring second-line treatment to achieve remission.[14] Numbers of evaluated clinical practice guidelines have failed in numerous respects, including not taking due account of the patient's viewpoint.[15]

Pertinent to the legitimacy of basic work in this sector, there are significant challenges to the reliability of the scientific principles and evidence behind the development of one of the most important references in the mental health sector – the *Diagnostic and Statistical Manual of Mental Disorders (DSM)*.[16] As an example of the imprecision involved, the very definition of depression has changed over time. It is now so broad that a formal published article in the *British Medical Journal* claims that it has resulted in over diagnosis and over treatment on an enormous scale.[17] Even some involved with the development of

DSM have later become critical of its direction. It is worthy to note that the co-author of this particular critical article is Allen Frances, who was the Chair of the DSM-IV Task Force, an earlier version of the DSM V.

The broad definition of depression reduces the likelihood of quality research and is so loose that, in everyday clinical practice, any general distress may be diagnosed as clinical depression.

Some researchers believe there is very little evidence of effectiveness of screening for depression in either average-risk or high-risk populations.[18] Screening tools are unable to clearly distinguish between the range and types of symptoms with which patients in distress present. For children and adolescents as well, there is concern that the screening process itself may in fact lead to over diagnosis.[19] Some American researchers believe that the unexamined assumptions and unintended consequences of questionnaire-based screening has serious consequences and may inadvertently become a driver of over diagnosis and over treatment, as well as taking away limited resources from those who need them most.[20]

The symptoms used to describe depression are so broad in screening tools that they are indistinguishable from a range of other general responses to distress, as well as from other potential clinical conditions such as substance abuse and physical health problems. Even researchers who are generally supportive of the mental disorder and treatment paradigm believe that 'screening is important, but it cannot be relied upon'.[21]

There have been challenges to the very idea of clinical depression for some time.[22] These include the fundamental concern around the biomedical idea that depressive states are brain disorders caused by chemical imbalances that can be corrected with disease-specific drugs.[23] Despite widespread faith in the potential of neuroscience to revolutionise mental health practice, the era of the biomedical model has been broadly characterised by a lack of clinical innovation and poor mental health outcomes. In addition, compounding the challenges of providing appropriate support for people in distress, the biomedical paradigm has profoundly affected clinical psychology via the adoption of drug trial methodology in psychotherapy research.[24] One of the criticisms levelled at the concept of depression as a clinical category is that the rationale for the category is built upon a circular argument:

> *The concept of depression is defined according to the symptoms of depression, which are in turn defined according to the concept of depression. Thus, it is impossible to be certain that the concept of depression maps onto any distinct disease entity, particularly since a diagnosis of depression can apply to anything from mild depression to depressive psychosis and depressive stupor, and overlap with several other categories of mental disorder including dysthymia, adjustment disorders, and anxiety disorders. Indeed, one of the consequences of the 'menu of symptoms' approach to diagnosing depression is that two people with absolutely no symptoms in common can both end up with the same diagnosis of depression. For this reason especially, the concept of depression has been charged with being little more than a socially constructed dustbin for all manner of human suffering.[25]*

Earlier evidence for the effectiveness of antidepressants helped the growth of the biomedical approach to diagnosis and treatment. However, that earlier evidence is now being seriously questioned – and there are those who believe that the current medical approach of diagnosing clinical depression and treatment with drugs is essentially baseless.[26] Indeed, a recent meta-analysis from the UK suggests that the diagnosis for clinical depression was only correct in 47% of cases presenting in primary care.[27]

There are a number of intersecting layers and dimensions of concern about the clinical category of depression:

> *The apparent increase in major depression results from: confusing those who are ill with those who share their symptoms; the surveying of symptoms out of context; the benefits that accrue from such a diagnosis to drug companies, researchers, and clinicians;*

and changing social constructions around sadness and distress. Standardized medical treatment of all these individuals is neither possible nor desirable.[28]

The rise of depression has been strongly driven by the development of antidepressants

Since the 1950s, both 'depression' and 'anxiety' have come to prominence as both medical constructs and general social concerns, and there is a wealth of research detailing the rise of depression, in particular, as a social phenomenon.[29] A brief look at the history of the rise of depression as a clinical category, and the key social and political dynamics that have underpinned it, is illuminating.

From times as early as the ancient Greeks, there was a broad concept of melancholia for general sadness and this included 'all forms of quiet insanity'. The term 'depression', used as a specific medical category, only began to appear in the 19th century.[30]

During the 1950s and 1960s, anxiety was the more common clinical mental health issue. Depression was considered a rare condition, and 'antidepressant' medications were mainly reserved for serious depressive conditions found in hospitalised patients.[31] Through the 1950s and 1960s, it was generally understood that stress was related to a 'diffuse and multifaceted array of psychic, somatic, and interpersonal problems' associated with the challenges of everyday life.[32]

The common psychological features of these problems include a mélange of symptoms involving nervousness, sadness, and malaise. The typical physical symptoms consist of headaches, fatigue, back pain, gastrointestinal complaints, and sleep and appetite difficulties, often accompanying struggles with interpersonal, financial, occupational, and health concerns.[33]

According to some researchers, during this time the concept of 'depression' barely existed, and 'antidepressant' medications were reserved mainly for serious depressive conditions found in hospitalised patients.[34]

From the early 1970s, and through the 1980s and 1990s, several interrelated dynamics facilitated the enormous rise of diagnosis for clinical depression and the prescription of antidepressants drugs on a huge scale across the world. These dynamics included the changing norms of psychiatric classification, increasing professional and political influence, and economic organisation and marketing. These all worked together so that toward the end of the 20th century the 'age of anxiety' became an 'age of depression'.[35]

The fundamental premise rationalising the treatment of depression with drugs is that, regardless of the harm associated with these drugs, antidepressants do *work* – that is, it is claimed that they achieve a reduction in depression. Presumably the risk of acknowledged side effects is considered to be worth it, with treatment plans inferring that patients are better off dealing with some side effects than continuing to suffer the symptoms that have been diagnosed as clinical depression. But the research is contradictory. While there is research that suggests some degree of efficacy for some antidepressants, there is also considerable research questioning whether these drugs actually do achieve the desired outcomes, and whether the research suggesting that they do is valid.

In the first instance, it is reasonable to think that antidepressant drugs can only work if there is a distinct state of depression that correlates with a brain analysis with which drugs can interact, to 'correct' the brain imbalance. Some recent research, published in 2018, challenges earlier research that suggests that antidepressants do work and that the drugs can 'cure' depression:

Contrary to the predominant interpretation we contend that antidepressants do not work in most patients, given that only 1 of 9 people benefit, whereas the remaining 8 are unnecessarily put at risk of adverse drug effects. To be clear, antidepressants can have strong mental and physical effects in some patients that may be considered helpful for some time but there is no evidence that the drugs can cure depression.[36]

It has been declared that the small advantage that antidepressants have over placebos in randomised control trials (RCTs) is easily accounted for by nonspecific psychological and pharmacologic effects.[37] Historically, the growth of Default Depression has been justified by research that suggested some effectiveness from antidepressant drug trials. And despite research that has strongly challenged the earlier work,[38] Default Depression continues to prevail.

To quote an article published in 2017 in *Frontiers of Psychiatry*, 'Methodological flaws, conflicts of interest, and scientific fallacies: Implications for the evaluation of antidepressants' efficacy and harm':

> *The strong reliance on industry-funded research results in an uncritical approval of antidepressants. Due to a number of important limitations and even outright flawed research methodology such as publication and reporting bias, unblinding of outcome assessors and concealment and recoding of serious adverse events, the efficacy of antidepressants is systematically overestimated, and harm is systematically underestimated.[39]*

The creation of the formal clinical diagnosis of depression

The publication of the *Diagnostic and Statistical Manual (DSM-III)* in 1980 radically changed the nature of psychiatric diagnoses by establishing a foundational principle that diagnostic criteria did not have to assume any particular causes of symptoms. A physician could now diagnose without empirical evidence of the cause and use their own interpretation of the patient's subjective description of 'symptoms'.[40]

This direction was further shored up when the modern concept of depression was written into the two key classification documents, *The ICD-10 Classification of Mental and Behavioral Disorders* and the fourth edition of the *Diagnostic and Statistical Manual of Mental Disorders (DSM-IV)* – both first published in the early 1990s. These classification systems are used worldwide and are important guides for clinical practice. The concept of depression was now understood to be 'essentially one of a clinical syndrome, defined by the presence of a number of clinical features, but not requiring a specific etiology [cause], and acknowledging the possibility of both psychological and biological causative factors'.[41] Again, this is a very broad and imprecise definition. These new definitions extended the parameters of clinical depression to encompass far more patients than any particular anxiety disorder.[42]

Past advocates and even key players in the development of the DSM have begun to acknowledge the poor science and unhelpful history of the development of the definition of clinical depression and the broader medicalising of human distress. Allen Frances, Chair of the DSM-IV Task Force (mentioned above) has written:

> *mislabeling everyday problems as mental illness has shocking implications for individuals and society: stigmatising a healthy person as mentally ill leads to unnecessary, harmful medications, the narrowing of horizons, misallocation of medical resources, and draining of the budgets of families and the nation. We also shift responsibility for our mental wellbeing away from our own naturally resilient and self-healing brains, which have kept us sane for hundreds of thousands of years, and into the hands of 'Big Pharma', who are reaping multi-billion-dollar profits.*[43]

The most recent DSM, DSM-5, published in 2013, has been described as creating 'the worst crisis in confidence in psychiatry in 40 years'.[44]

A fundamental consideration for diagnosis in the clinical mental health setting is the distinction between a dimensional view and a categorical view. The current major classification systems, DSM and the International Classification of Diseases (ICD), published by the World Health Organization, are based on the categorical approach. The categorical approach is a dichotomous approach – and can be decidedly unhelpful. It determines that a person either does or doesn't have a mental disorder. Within this framework, there is little room to consider the current degree or intensity of stress, or of the current state having a place in an overall process of healing. The categorical approach also provides little practical guidance for mental health professionals in considering fundamental issues around the extent of psychological or emotional distress.[45] There have also been critiques of the ambiguous symptomology on which the classification is based.[46]

The criticisms of the specific condition of clinical depression sit within broader concerns about defining and categorising mental disorders generally. There are dangers of the categorical approach to psychological or emotional distress:

> The use of psychiatric diagnosis increases stigma, does not aid treatment decisions, is associated with worsening long-term prognosis for mental health problems, and imposes Western beliefs about mental distress on other cultures. Alternative evidence-based models for organising effective mental health care are available.[47]

There are similar concerns expressed about several aspects of this issue, including that the diagnosis of mental disorders may diminish practitioner–client relationships.[48]

Complementing these concerns, another paper published in *Frontiers of Psychiatry* describes several related challenges and offers a scathing critique of mental health assessment:

> We demonstrate substantial inconsistency in the inclusion and emphasis of symptoms assessed within disorders as well as considerable symptom overlap across disorder-specific tools … The consequence of this inconsistent and heterogeneous assessment landscape is that it hinders clinical diagnosis and treatment and frustrates understanding of the social, environmental, and biological factors that contribute to mental health symptoms and disorders. Altogether, it underscores the need for standardized assessment tools that are more disorder agnostic and span the full spectrum of mental health symptoms to aid the understanding of underlying etiologies and the discovery of new treatments for psychiatric dysfunction.[49]

Rising rates of diagnosis of clinical depression and anxiety disorders

Default Depression is a global trend. Over the last several decades, there has been an enormous increase in both the diagnoses of clinical depression and the prescribing of antidepressants across much of the Western world.[50]

While there are more and more treatment cases of clinical depression carried out, the number of people with depression is rising, not falling. According to the WHO, the total estimated number of people living with depression increased by 18.4% between 2005 and 2015.[51]

Rates of anxiety disorder are also rising across the globe. The total estimated number of people living with anxiety disorders in the world was 264 million in 2015. This reflects a 14.9% increase since 2005.[52]

A major report from the insurance industry in the US gives an account of huge increases in diagnoses of clinical depression in just the last few years; since just 2013, diagnoses of major depression have risen dramatically by 33%, rising even faster among millennials (up 47%) and adolescents (up 47% for boys and 65% for girls).[53]

There is a similar story in the United Kingdom. There has been a general increase in the last few years. In 2014, 19.7% of people in the UK aged 16 and over showed symptoms of anxiety or depression – a 1.5% increase from 2013. This percentage was higher among females (22.5%) than males (16.8%). There have been even greater increases in diagnoses of depression among workers where rates of moderate to extreme anxiety and depression have soared by 30.5% since 2013.[54]

There has also been a general rise in the rate of diagnosis of clinical depression in Australia in recent years with a notable rise in the incidence of depression and anxiety among those aged 15 to 34. In 2017, 20.1% of females and 11.2% of males in this age group reported being affected by these conditions compared to 12.8% of females and 6.1% of males in 2009.[55] Mental illness is also the most reported serious illness among Australians aged under 55.[56]

Rates of mental disorder in children are also very high; the 2015 second Australian childhood and adolescent survey of mental health and wellbeing reported that in the 12 months prior to the survey around one in seven (13.9%) children and adolescents aged 4–17 years experienced a mental disorder. This is equivalent to an estimated 560,000 Australian children and adolescents.[57]

There is an enormous economic cost that comes with this. The Royal Australian and New Zealand Collage of Psychiatrists estimated the cost burden of serious mental illness, including opioid dependence, in Australia at $98.8 billion in 2016.[58] While much of this covers the general intervention-level costs of mental health treatment, such as hospitalisation and staffing, much of this treatment activity and cost is targeted at depression and anxiety rather than severe psychiatric disorders because a substantial number of patients diagnosed with severe 'mental disorders' are those with depressive and anxiety disorders. In fact, the number of these patients far outweigh those with schizophrenia and severe bipolar disorder combined.[59]

It should be noted that while the data quoted here on rising rates of depression are publicly available, it is important to maintain a crucial distinction – these data refer to rising rates of *clinical depression*. Rising rates of clinical depression are a result of more diagnoses – and this should not be interpreted as a measure of the general wellbeing of the community. As a contrasting interpretation, this book asserts that the rise in rates of depression can be seen to a large extent as *situational distress*, misdiagnosed as clinical depression.

Recent media reports about the sector in the context of COVID-19 paint a similar picture, describing large increases in mental health claims including specific references to depression and anxiety diagnoses.[60]

Stigmatisation persists

The stigma of mental illness is a major issue. Despite large amounts of money spent on campaigns designed to reduce the stigma associated with mental illness, stigmatisation prevails and is still a major burden on people diagnosed with a mental disorder. As described, diagnosing someone with clinical depression is not a minor issue; the diagnostic label is a permanent stamp in that patient's medical history. They are likely to need to disclose this in any number of social circumstances, such as applying for a new job, or when undergoing a legal or judicial process. In the UK, the Mental Health Foundation reports that nearly nine out of ten people with mental health problems say that stigma and discrimination have a negative effect on their lives.[61]

A 2016 meta-analysis revealed that stigmatisation due to mental illness is a universal and disabling problem, and that it is present among both children and adults.[62] According to this analysis, this prevalence of mental illness stigma exists despite large-scale initiatives to reduce the stigmatisation of mental illness, which the authors describe as 'disappointing'. A fundamental dynamic in the creation of stigma is the very process of applying diagnostic labels, such as the all-too-common label of clinical depression, which may in fact greatly exacerbate the experience of psychological/emotional challenges:

Stigma can greatly exacerbate the experience of mental illness. Diagnostic classification frequently used by clinical social workers may intensify this stigma by enhancing the public's sense of 'groupness' and 'differentness' when perceiving people with mental illness. The homogeneity assumed by stereotypes may lead mental health professionals and the public to view individuals in terms of their diagnostic labels. The stability of stereotypes may exacerbate notions that people with mental illness do not recover. Several strategies may diminish the unintended effects of diagnosis. Dimensional approaches to diagnosis may not augment stigma in the same manner as classification. Moreover, regular interaction with people with mental illness and focusing on recovery may diminish the stigmatizing effects of diagnosis.[63]

Research published in 2018 clearly shows that the stigma round mental health is still a major concern, with impacts on people throughout different sectors of the community.

Mental illness stigma is as a major obstacle to wellbeing among people with mental illness (PWMI). According to findings from the most recent nationally representative study of public attitudes toward mental illness in the US, only 42% of Americans aged 18–24 believe PWMI can be successful at work, 26% believe that others have a caring attitude toward PWMI, and 25% believe that PWMI can recover from their illness … A robust body of evidence demonstrates that PWMI experience discrimination in nearly every domain of their lives, including employment … housing … and medical care … Experiences of stigma are associated with increased symptom severity … decreased treatment seeking … and treatment non-adherence …[64]

Stigmatisation of mental illness in the workplace is common.[65] Research published in 2020 into workplace mental health in the UK shows that stigma is still a major obstruction to improving personal wellbeing:

Stigma and fear remain the two most common blockers to talking about mental wellbeing openly, both within the workplace and within our society.[66]

There are similar concerns about stigma and discrimination in the workplace in Australia.[67]

In short, there are a number of complex social dynamics that add to the burden of the stigmatisation of mental illness.[68] Despite significant funding to destigmatise mental illness, there is a clear need to address how the stigma of mental health also manifests more widely as prejudice against people with mental illness.[69] The terrible irony in the stigmatisation of mental health is that it is the very system of formally diagnosing (labelling) people with mental health conditions that differentiates people and creates the circumstances for judgemental attitudes.

Marketing of antidepressant drugs – depression versus anxiety

The enormous global pharmaceutical industry has been a key driver in the extraordinary rise of depression as a medical and social issue. The clinical categorisation of depression in the early 1990s dramatically broadened the opportunity to apply newly developed antidepressant drugs. This came to dominate the treatment of a range of patient symptoms, including depression, but also various anxiety disorders, and other conditions.[70]

Advertising by the pharmaceutical industry took advantage of the new opportunity to promote antidepressant drugs; and gradually, over the last decades of the 20th century, diagnoses for depression overtook diagnoses for anxiety.[71] By the early 2000s, the term depression was applied to a very broad range of symptoms and disparate experiences of anguish or suffering. Pharmaceutical companies promoted their new products to physicians and psychiatrists as drugs that treated a variety of nonspecific complaints, including anxiety, tension, depression and mental stress. Adding to the concerns and questions around scientific validity, the pharmaceutical industry deliberately fed this general ambiguity and vagueness with advertisements that typically connected the most general symptoms of depression from the DSM's descriptions – sadness, fatigue, sleeplessness, and the like – with common situations such as dealing with unruly children, traffic jams, demanding bosses and housekeeping.[72]

Pharmaceutical companies began marketing their antidepressants through medical and psychiatric journals as well as directly to physicians and, later, consumers.[73] Treatment statistics during the 1970s reflected the growing interest in depression. During the first half of that decade, the management of depression became as common as that of anxiety.[74] This was to such an extent that, 'Between 1987 and 1997, the proportion of the US population receiving outpatient treatment for conditions called "depression" increased by more than 300 per cent'.[75] And by 2000, 10% of the population was using antidepressants, the best-selling category of drugs of any sort in the United States.[76]

There had been a significant shift in the medical industry's thinking around psychological and emotional challenges. These difficulties were now specifically being called depression, replacing generalised terms such as anxiety, tension, nerves or stress.[77]

Biomedical paradigm – the development of the biological mental disorder

Establishing the paradigm of a biological basis for mental disorder has been a complementary and integral trend to the dynamics described above, and a major factor in the rise of clinical depression. Across the globe, research, diagnosis and treatment for mental health now largely sits within this paradigm.

The biomedical model posits that mental disorders are brain diseases and emphasizes pharmacological treatment to target presumed biological abnormalities. A biologically focused approach to science, policy, and practice has dominated the American healthcare system for more than three decades.[78]

The rise of the biomedical paradigm was strategic. By the late 1970s, biologically oriented researchers had joined the fight against psychosocial research in general, and more specifically – and strategically importantly – within the United States' National Institute of Mental Health (NIMH).[79] This lobbying influenced the NIMH to redirect social research to focus more directly on the biological underpinnings of, and treatments for, specific mental disorders. This lobbying was so successful that in 1982, the US Congress ordered the NIMH to stop its support of social research.[80]

Complementing this, during the 1970s, US government regulators began to more stringently enforce the legislative requirement, dating from 1962, that drug companies target the marketing of their products to particular biomedical conditions.[81] Whatever the original intention of the legislation may have been, it had now become a powerful factor in the rise of antidepressants.

The success of the biomedical model has become pervasive across the planet, and the resultant sales of antidepressants staggering. There are consistent global trends; business journals show how marketing strategies for antidepressants are considered as a global market, with market dynamic and market trends considered within a global context.[82] By 2018, the antidepressant drug market was valued at US$13.69 billion.[83] Australia is a part of this global exercise. We are a part of the marketing strategies described above and the Therapeutic Goods Administration (Australia's main drug regulation body) has a well-established working relationship with the FDA from the US.[84]

Anxiety is on the rise again

There is evidence that the marketing from pharmaceutical companies has once again turned to anxiety. The NIMH reports that '[a]nxiety disorders are the most common mental illness in the US, affecting 40 million adults in the United States age 18 and older, or 18.1% of the population every year'.[85] In Australia, key mental health organisations, such as Beyond Blue, have increased their messaging around anxiety disorder. For example: 'Everyone feels anxious from time to time. When anxious feelings don't go away, happen without any particular reason or make it hard to cope with daily life it may be the sign of an anxiety condition.' Language such as this medicalises anxiety.[86]

To feel anxious is an important biological state and should not be presumed to be pathological. It is important for safety; it is important for nurturing; it is important for discipline and achievement.

Anxiety itself is a normal physiological response to a stressful situation. Often described as being nervous, worried or on edge ... physiological symptoms of anxiety may include a pounding heart, shortness of breath, dizziness, trembling and the sensation of 'butterflies in the stomach'.[87]

As with depression, the clinical definition of anxiety attempts to distinguish between 'normal anxiety' and 'GAD – Generalised Anxiety Disorder'. However:

The diagnosis of generalised anxiety disorder is a distraction of no value. It is highly unreliable, co-occurring with many other disorders of firmer diagnostic status …[88]

The attempts to distinguish anxiety – a perfectly normal physiological response to a stressful situation – from the idea of a formalised clinical anxiety disorder fall into the same sorts of semantic and logic problems as trying to distinguish different types of depression.[89] Compounding the often unhelpful clinical approach to both depression and anxiety, the symptoms of both are largely the same as each other, and indeed, in some clinical definitions, 'depression' is listed as a symptom of anxiety disorder.[90]

There is conjecture that the promotion of anxiety as an illness is happening in part because it is becoming increasingly difficult and expensive to develop new antidepressants.[91] However, for the purposes of marketing antidepressants, the category 'anxiety' sometimes includes 'depression' and the symptoms of the two categories are almost identical – meaning that there is room to market the existing drugs to a new cohort.

Generalised anxiety disorder symptoms include:
- Feeling restless, wound-up, or on-edge
- Being easily fatigued
- Having difficulty concentrating; mind going blank
- Being irritable
- Having muscle tension
- Difficulty controlling feelings of worry
- Having sleep problems, such as difficulty falling or staying asleep, restlessness, or unsatisfying sleep

Treatment

Antidepressants

Antidepressants are used to treat depression, but they can also be helpful for treating anxiety disorders.

Figure 3. Generalised anxiety disorder symptoms,
from the National Institute of Mental Health in the US[92]

The last point is of a particular concern for diagnosing children with mental disorders in Australia, especially with the newly intensified marketing of anxiety as mental disorder and the targeting of the education sector for this purpose by key mental health organisations such as Beyond Blue. There are an increasing number of organisations delivering mental health training in schools. As described earlier, there are already 115,482 children on antidepressants in Australia.[93]

Studying the history of 'clinical depression' reveals its rise from a minor medical matter to one of the most common health-related issues, and one of the most common reasons for prescribing drugs as treatment. This rise has happened in just a few decades, and is related to the deliberate marketing of the concept of a specific clinical category of depression, along with the idea that this is treatable with drugs.

Chapter 3

The role of the mental health sector

It is no coincidence that there is a significant upward trend in suicide deaths, diagnoses of depression and prescribing of antidepressants *and* economic cost because these phenomena are integrally related.

Despite the well-meaning efforts of many activists at the community level, the influence of those leading the current approach is so comprehensive that the funding directed into communities is generally conditional on following a limited range of program types. Common examples are celebrity ambassadors talking publicly about their depression, postvention support being presented as suicide 'prevention', and mental health training programs that essentially promulgate the biomedical approach. This sort of activity is not necessarily a bad thing in its own right, but these activities are funded at the exclusion of others that may be more effective, particularly in the context of a local community.

There is plenty of anecdotal evidence from community activists around the country describing how their requests for a different approach are disregarded by the sector. Mt Druitt Shed (The Shed) in Western Sydney is an example of where a different approach has been supported.[1] This well-established community-level activity includes a range of human services, beyond the health/mental health sector, integrated into the support provided for the different needs of people in distress. Housing, finance, employment and legal services all have important supportive roles for the clients of The Shed. This sort of initiative should be a priority for further development and replication around the country as an appropriate model of suicide prevention.

Another good example of operating effectively comes from the Central Coast of NSW. When the mental health/suicide prevention sector offered no financial support to curb regular suicide deaths from the Mooney Mooney Bridge, the Central Coast Suicide Safety Network drew on road safety funding to design and build a barrier fence on the bridge.[2] This made an immediate impact, significantly reducing the suicide deaths from that hotspot, and follow-up analysis of local data showed it was not replaced by a substitute location.

A comprehensive analysis by Melissa Raven in her award-winning PhD thesis highlights the enormous influence of a small number of key individuals and organisations in raising the profile of depression as a key mental health issue in Australia through the last couple of decades of the 20th century and into this century.[3]

Raven and her colleagues, in a paper published in 2020 in the *Frontiers in Psychiatry*, describe examples of how prominent mental health organisations and key opinion leaders have influenced prescribing trends, resulting in the rapid increase in the use of antidepressants between 2009 and 2018. Referring to the relationship between antidepressants and suicide the authors maintain: 'There have been numerous examples of these influential organisations and individuals incorrectly interpreting or reporting evidence.' The paper offers a damning critique of Australia's peak body on suicide prevention, and gives a detailed description of the role Suicide Prevention Australia (SPA) have made in the increase in antidepressant use, including: making unreferenced claims, misrepresenting the findings of one important review, ignoring key findings of another important review and minimising the importance of the US Federal Drug Administration (FDA) and the Australian Therapeutic Goods Administration (TGA) suicidality warnings.[4]

Complementing this analysis, Martin Whitely's recent book also describes the key role that high-profile individuals and organisations in the mental health/suicide prevention sector have played in promulgating the illness paradigm in mental health, its focus on depression implying a clinical disorder.[5]

Depression and the mental health narrative in Australia

This focus on depression in Australia has corresponded with similar campaigns in the US and the UK in the 1980s and 1990s. These international campaigns helped lead to the development of the National Depression Awareness Campaign, launched in 1994 by the Mental Health Foundation of Australia.[6] This campaign was designed to educate the public that depression is 'serious, common and treatable', and significantly influenced the initiation and development of Beyond Blue, still a leading player in the sector.[7]

As outlined in the Introduction, there is ambiguity around the terms 'mental health' and the 'mental health system'. The mental health/suicide prevention sector is in fact much broader than the mental health system, which generally refers to the specific institutions and personnel of the clinical mental health aspect of the health system. But there is significant overlap between the leadership and experts of the mental health system and the broader mental health/suicide prevention sector. And concern is growing about the effectiveness of the mental health/suicide prevention sector, and the mental health system itself. In Victoria, the recent Royal Commission into Victoria's Mental Health System has highlighted this. In the Commission's *Final Report*, Victoria's mental health system is strongly criticised (and many of these criticisms also apply to the broader mental health/suicide prevention sector). Briefly, they include:

- *There is a patchwork of services that do not reflect local needs.*
- *Services are poorly integrated.*
- *The perspectives and experiences of people with lived experience of mental illness or psychological distress are overlooked.*
- *Communities and places do not adequately support good mental health and wellbeing.*
- *Some groups face further barriers.*

- *Housing instability can compound mental illness.*
- *Stigma and discrimination are ever present.*
- *Good mental health and wellbeing are not given priority.*
- *The system's foundations need reform.*
- *Regulation and oversight is complex and unclear.*
- *Dignity is often disregarded and human rights are breached.*
- *The system is antiquated.*[8]

These concerns, recently expressed in Australia and internationally, are about the fundamental conceptualisation of mental health and the mental health system. A 2020 article from Sam Timimi in the online psychiatric magazine, Mad in the UK puts some of the concerns into sharp focus:

Mainstream mental health services are a disaster. The problem isn't under-funding or the scale of the mental health challenge in society. It isn't social media, stigma, lack of education, lack of doctors or therapists. The problem is the dominant ideology. It's the concepts of mental health, mental 'wellness', mental illness, and mental disorder that pervade our societies.

It's the way we have come to talk and think about mental health. It's the narratives that the public are exposed to, day in day out, popularising a jaundiced, scientifically illiterate idea that we know what sort of a 'thing' mental disorder is, that it is widespread, and needs diagnosing, so that effective treatments can be provided. It's the endless expansion and commercialisation of so-called psychiatric diagnoses, so that they operate as lucrative brands rather than legitimate categories that help build knowledge and improve clinical practice.[9]

Even the Royal Commission itself was not without pointed criticism, including criticism of the Commission's stated purpose and terms of reference.[10] Others asserted there was general confusion in the Commission's documentation around issues such as improving the mental health of the population and the determinants of mental health.

What we describe as mental health, and the mental health system, needs wholesale reconsideration, along with new leadership, to ensure integrity to the critique and revision of the broader sector and the system.

Political and economic influences on the mental health narrative in Australia

Pharmaceutical companies have had a central role in the development of the growth of the current approach to suicide prevention and mental health. Several respected researchers give detailed accounts of the role the pharmaceutical industry plays in mental health.[11]

Early in the Australian historical context of the rise of the narrative of the mental health/illness paradigm, and particularly depression as a public health and general public issue, the *Depression Awareness Journal* was funded by two pharmaceutical companies and distributed to Australian doctors by the Mental Health Foundation of Australia to complement the general community awareness-raising of depression.[12]

In Australia the standout organisation in mental health has been Beyond Blue – formerly featuring a telling by-line, the 'National Depression Initiative'.[13] Perhaps more than any other organisation, Beyond Blue has been instrumental in the rise of depression as a core issue in the public perception of mental health in Australia. They have proudly publicised their role in the increasing numbers of diagnoses of depression and anxiety as mental illness. A Beyond Blue media release from 2014 shows clearly their intention in this disturbing trend:

> *beyondblue has welcomed new research that shows the remarkable growth of treatment rates for mental health conditions in Australia in recent years … The study by Professor Harvey Whiteford and colleagues found the treatment rate for mental disorders in Australia soared from 37% in 2006–07 to 46% in 2009–10, a growth the authors believe has not been seen anywhere else in the world.*
>
> *beyondblue CEO Kate Carnell AO said the increase was due partly to the good work of mental health organisations such as*

beyondblue ... 'The fact that more people are seeking treatment for mental health conditions such as depression and anxiety is wonderful news,' she said.[14]

While it has more recently broadened its focus to include promoting the medicalisation of anxiety as a disorder, for most of its 20-year history, it has been focused on depression. Beyond Blue is now a huge organisation in its own right, with an annual surplus in the multi-millions of dollars.[15] It is a key influencer in the development of workplace mental health policy and practice and has developed a range of products and services that perpetuate the focus on depression as well as the organisation's predominance in the sector. Beyond Blue has a significant commercial interest in mental health, particularly in the workplace, through their own commercial activity, as well as through issuing licensing rights to other commercial ventures, such as workplace mental health training. In the early 2000s, Beyond Blue established a model of workplace mental health training that has heavily influenced the culture of workplace mental health since.[16] Workplace-based mental health/ suicide prevention activity, especially mental health training, is now a huge business in its own right – and largely reiterates the current illness paradigm. For example, core aspects of training programs promise participants they will learn to identify depression and to know about appropriate treatment.[17]

The substantial government and philanthropic funding directed into the mental health sector has been a major economic and business benefit to organisations like Beyond Blue, and has been described as 'funding mental health brands rather than mental health care'.[18]

Despite strong challenges to Beyond Blue on several fronts across its history, the organisation has stood firm, and continues to disregard evidence and expertise that challenges the validity of its approach.[19] There have been reports of questionable public commentary from senior personnel, as well as serious discordant relationships among its senior personnel.[20]

Business interests

Beyond Blue is strongly favoured by government and in a crucial move toward further entrenching depression as a standard institutional approach to issues around psychological and emotional wellbeing, governments now outsource much of the administration of government activity in this sector, with Beyond Blue featuring heavily in government literature and in a range of key activities. As such, governments effectively endorse Beyond Blue as representing the government's position on mental health and suicide prevention.[21]

The vast funding now directed into the mental health/suicide prevention sector has effectively protected the business interests of key players, but this politicising of the issue has been challenged:

> There is a great deal of misinformation about suicide and the causes of suicide which has helped to establish mindsets and myths about suicide and how to prevent it … The uncritical assessment of evidence and misinformation are responsible for the politicisation of suicide prevention policy development. Politicisation of suicide prevention, in turn, has made all the actors involved part of the problem, rather than the solution.[22]

The former Prime Minister Julia Gillard is now Chair of Beyond Blue. She has developed a strong media presence as a powerful advocate for anxiety as a mental disorder.[23] From 2018, Beyond Blue has been further pushing the institutionalisation of mental health into the school system.[24] This more recent focus on anxiety is a grave concern. The terrible consequences of misdiagnosis and inappropriate prescribing of potentially harmful drugs to children, including for anxiety, have been illustrated in a number of recent media reports, and this deliberate push into the education sector is in stark contrast to concerns recently stated by the United Nations:

> Overmedicalization is especially harmful to children, and global trends to medicalize complex psychosocial and public health issues in childhood should be addressed with a stronger political will.[25]

The number of children who will now be misdiagnosed and prescribed potentially harmful drugs as a result of this campaign by Beyond Blue is of great concern.

While Beyond Blue is the biggest organisation pushing the focus on depression and the paradigm of illness in the Australian context, it is not alone. Other not-for-profit organisations, including academic institutions and religious organisations, often seek to partner with Beyond Blue in research and program delivery; partnerships that serve Beyond Blue's strategic business interests by enabling the broadest possible dissemination of their brand and approach.

Together these key organisations have strongly and overtly influenced the uptake of the policies and practices that perpetuate Default Depression across all sectors, particularly the corporate sector. They provide a range of services and products including training programs, facilitated strategic planning and policy development. This makes perfect commercial sense; corporate organisations have mandatory budgets for training and the related continuing quality improvement activity, which has also grown markedly as a strong corporate trend across the Western world over the last three to four decades. It means there are huge amounts of money available for workplace mental health training.

The medicalisation process is fully integrated into the mental health/suicide prevention sector and the training it provides. In earlier promotional material for the workplace, Beyond Blue clearly equates depression and anxiety with illness:

> *Established in 2000, initially by the Commonwealth and Victorian Governments, beyondblue is a bipartisan initiative of the Australian, State and Territory Governments, with the key goals of raising community awareness about depression and anxiety and reducing stigma associated with the illnesses.*
>
> *Our five priorities are:*
> 1. *Increasing community awareness of depression, anxiety and related disorders and addressing associated stigma.*

2   *Providing people living with depression and anxiety and their
carers with information on these illnesses and effective treatment
options and promoting their needs and experiences with policy
makers and healthcare service providers.*

Like Beyond Blue, the Black Dog Institute has also had a major
role in pushing the illness paradigm in workplace training. The Black
Dog Mental Health Toolkit, for example, is dominated by references to
mental illness and they are proud to be

*a global pioneer in the identification, prevention and treatment of
mental illness.* [26]

Suicide prevention activity in Australia now very generally echoes
the paradigm of illness with its focus on clinical mental disorders,
particularly depression. We need to challenge this culture of
medicalisation. As M. Louis Ruffalo stated in 2014:

*The medicalisation of suicide is not without consequence: it distorts
our understanding of suicide, leads to the dissemination of false
information about suicide, and contributes further to the stigma
surrounding suicide and mental illness.*[27]

The culture of medicalisation has hindered suicide prevention
efforts:

*A significant consequence of an eagerness to diagnose mental illness
in people experiencing psychological distress, unfortunately turns up
in the field of suicide prevention, and may well be putting people at
greater risk of suicide. This is because suicide prevention initiatives,
preoccupied with detection of 'mental illness' – such as depression –
often overlook and fail to address forms of distress that don't
constitute any kind of illness or disorder, and yet which can result
in suicidal ideation (thoughts preoccupied with suicide) and suicide.*

*The current mental illness narrative evident in mental health
literacy messaging and commentary on suicide prevention has
tended to reinforce the idea that suicide should, in most cases, be*

considered to be the result of mental illness or disorder. However, evidence does not support this claim. Whilst conditions like major depression may sometimes be implicated in cases of suicidal ideation and death by suicide and are an important consideration in the design of appropriate preventative measures, this should not be considered license to assume an association between the two that is simply unsupported. Limiting preventive strategies to those built upon the unfounded presumption of mental illness or disorder will simply not help many, perhaps the majority, of those at risk of suicide.[28]

Even when evaluations, including fully independent evaluations, measure poor performance by leading national, government-funded mental health organisations, there appears to be no will among the current leadership to challenge the place and funding of these organisations; the very well-funded headspace program is a good example of this.[29] The *Medical Journal of Australia* published an article in 2022, 'Latest evidence casts further doubt on the effectiveness of headspace';[30] Australian media reported on this and headspace was described as an 'abject failure'[31] and as the 'McDonalds version of healthcare'.[32] The *Sydney Morning Herald* article reported that leading mental health experts had described heasdspace as 'an unfolding disaster within Australia's national youth mental health service'. Matt Noffs, chief executive of the Ted Noffs Foundation, was particularly cutting:

This is what happens when we don't spend time looking at the evidence, when we don't think about good governance and structure. It's one thing if it was a corporation but this is meant to be saving young people's lives.

Key individual 'experts' are favoured as media spokespersons, and highly celebrated personalities representing these key organisations have continued to push the focus on mental disorder; for example, the unfounded and thoroughly discredited notion that depression is involved in 90% of all suicide deaths.[33]

The business of delivering workplace training programs in suicide prevention and mental health now constitutes an enormous commercial activity in its own right; workplace training in Australia is a multi-billion dollar per annum industry.[34] Much of this is spent on mental health through literally thousands of workplace mental health training programs delivered every year.[35] The mental health sector has a major role delivering much of the mental health training conducted in the workplace. These programs are designed and delivered by organisations that maintain their market share and activity by perpetuating the current approach. They are now part of a systemic, bureaucratised approach to workplace stress that is further pushing the boundaries of the mental illness narrative. Large numbers of distressed workers are being directed into a narrow Default Depression pathway built around identifying, diagnosing and treating depression and/or anxiety, irrespective of the cause of the distress.

Also prevalent in workplace mental health training is the theme of resilience. A simple Google search will show just how commonplace this now is. And this means big business. Despite the extensive spread and current popularity of resilience in mental health training, there is a good deal of useful critique about this topic. A recent article in the *Guardian* describes resilience training as 'pop-psychology', and that:

At its worst, the resilience imperative is an offensive, exclusionary narrative that blames individuals for their predicament. Encouraging us to internalise, rather than question, the dominant logic of neoliberal values and the structural inequalities and social determinants that contribute to poor mental health ...[36]

Other concerns include that some managers may offer this training as a solution to a difficult situation just to avoid conflict.[37]

Perhaps of even greater concern is the spread of resilience training into the education system. A browse of the many resilience-training programs for schools shows the same emphasis on individual resilience without consideration of the social context of distressed schoolchildren. The general pop-psychology approach is evident. One high-profile program advertises on the home page of their website that its training program can help teachers to 'Energise, refocus and develop wellbeing in your students in 5 minutes'.[38]

The role of media

The different media are used strategically by key organisations in the mental health/suicide prevention sector to ensure the mental illness narrative and Default Depression are as deeply embedded into the structure of our community as possible, including as formal workplace policy. The workplace is hit with broad-scale messaging on mental health on morning television in the tearoom, to email memos from HR on workplace mental health as soon as the work computer is opened.

Government outsources the responsibility for the narrative on depression and anxiety to the very organisations who have built considerable commercial activity around depression and anxiety – and media in turn present representatives from these organisations to the community as the experts and authorities.

Quite apart from the commercial media's part in promoting and advertising well-funded mental health programs such as R U OK?, the national broadcaster ABC perpetuates the mental illness narrative too. In his book *Overprescribing Madness*, Martin Whitely describes how a 'particularly disappointing aspect of our national debate on mental health has been our national broadcaster's uncritical promotion of Professors McGorry and Hickie as authoritative, independent, trustworthy mental health gurus'.[39] In fact, it is some of these high-profile 'experts' and advocates who have been instrumental in perpetuating the paradigm of illness.

Publishing of research papers and expert opinion editorials through scientific and medical journals is a crucially important aspect of media and information dissemination. As the scientific journals are presumed to be sound in their science, broader media tends to refer uncritically to these sources as a part of journalistic inquiry and analysis for topical issues. In the case of Default Depression, general media play their part in perpetuating the ongoing confusion and unresolved issues within the broader debate around distress and what constitutes appropriate support. The publishing of some of this research material without criticism then effectively endorses the current approach. John Ashfield and I have written on this topic before:

> *The current approach by the media to the issues of suicide and 'mental health' is clearly dominated by a focus on the present conceptualisation of depression ... by the 'experts' and high-profile personalities who represent and promote this focus. Journalists tend to turn to a very select few to obtain opinions on suicide and mental health issues; consequently, the content of reporting and commentary is nearly always informed by the mental illness ideology.*
>
> *We need to encourage the development of a team of more incisive and critical journalists, interested to pursue a broader and more useful perspective on these issues, and one that breaks free of the facile thinking about depression and other 'disorders'.*
>
> *The mass media and those who have significant roles in public and organisational communication, can also assist the process of necessary change by becoming familiar with the new language now being proposed in the Situational Approach. This is crucial to ensuring that the broad spectrum of common human experience of distress of one sort or another, is not unnecessarily named and defined as 'mental illness' or 'mental disorder'; terms that are at best unhelpful, at worst harmful. Adopting new and better language is vitally important if we are to progress toward more effective suicide prevention and effective mental health literacy initiatives that promote the psychological wellbeing and mental health of individuals and our community.[40]*

The media too, must be held accountable for their role in Default Depression. They need to consider a broader range of evidence and experts before presenting information to the community. They need to show editorial integrity in the messages they offer as paid advertising. And they need to be prepared to publish articles that challenge, rather than compound, the current approach.

Chapter 4

Mental health in the workplace: Default Depression in organisational policy and practice

The policies and practices of Default Depression are not confined to the health and human services sectors. This phenomenon has spread throughout our community, particularly as formalised organisational policy and practice, over the last several decades.

Default Depression now pervades our day-to-day lives. Men, women and children who may be distressed are directed onto a pathway that leads to a diagnosis of mental disorder. It has become institutionalised in organisational culture, policy and practice across industries and sectors (including the workplace), schools and higher education, not-for-profits, entertainment and sport.

Governments at all levels sanction and promote this through policy and substantial funding allocation, and energetically partner with businesses and employers to make mental health a priority,[1] what is now known as 'workplace mental health' (WMH). The medicalisation of distress is promoted strongly through workplace training, to 'identify' a stressed person, and presume them to be depressed (implying a clinically diagnosable depression).[2] Whether or not the distressed person has a history of mental disorder, and whether or not the stress is the result of difficulties completely outside the individual's own making is largely irrelevant to this process.

The institutionalisation of the default response to distress in the workplace has had an enormous impact on workplace health and safety. Globally, mental disorders have now displaced musculoskeletal conditions as the predominant reason for illness-related absences and work incapacity.[3]

As a consequence, there are escalating numbers of diagnoses for workplace mental disorders (commonly clinical depression) and a large percentage of all sickness absence certified by GPs is due to common mental disorders.[4] In Australia there has also been dramatic increase in the proportion of the working age population receiving Disability Support Pension for psychiatric conditions.[5] As a consequence of this, and as described in a recent report by the Financial Services Council of Australia and KPMG, the escalating cost of worker compensation is significantly impacting the economic viability of the life insurance industry itself.[6] In 2020, the life insurance industry outlined its concerns about this issue in response to the federal government's *Draft Report on the Social & Economic Benefits of Improving Mental Health.*[7]

While some within the industry are attempting to provide appropriate support for distressed workers, the general framework and practices of workplace mental health still abide by the biomedical approach. For example, calls to include the provision of clinical treatment for all mental health-related workers' compensation claims, while perhaps well-intentioned, would further entrench the biomedical, individualising paradigm,[8] and create a corresponding increase of mental health as a proportion of GPs' workload.[9]

The contradiction here, from an industrial relations perspective, is that a significant percentage of workers believe that workplace conditions play a role in their distress.[10]

Across a broad range of settings, common human behaviours and feelings in response to stressful situations are 'identified' according to workplace policy, literature and training; these behaviours and feelings are then interpreted as symptomatic of a mental disorder, typically clinical depression. Authorities such as human resources personnel and school counsellors intervene and recommend or direct people, including school-age children, to visit a GP to determine or confirm a mental disorder. Following diagnosis, these 'patients' are now generally treated with antidepressants.

Diagnosis of mental disorder is often required for workplace support

The debate around the development of appropriate workplace mental health policy and practice is dominated by the current narrative around mental illness, that is, that the worker's distress is attributable to a diagnosable mental disorder. There have been attempts to consider the broader context of the causes of stress; for example, the recent paper from the Financial Services Council of Australia and KPMG discusses workplace distress in the life insurance sector and the role of psychosocial factors in this distress.[11] The typical workplace mental health training, resources and support, however, take little or no consideration of the causal correlates of the distress.

The typical formal workplace process involving distressed workers includes making insurance claims for work-related mental health conditions.[12] These claims are made to support the distressed worker, however, typical insurance industry literature, such as the following from MLC Insurance, advises distressed workers to engage with a GP *as the first step*:

> *There are a number of tactics to manage anxiety and depression, including counselling and medication.*
>
> *The first thing to do, however, is to seek help from your doctor, who can then advise on the best course of action.*[13]

A typical part of this process is developing a Mental Health Treatment Plan, with the presumption that clinical depression or anxiety disorder is fundamental to the problem.[14]

Medicalising workplace distress and making insurance claims against this as mental disorder is happening on a massive scale. In Australia, work-related mental health conditions are the second most common cause of workers' compensation.[15] And it is GPs who have a key role in decision-making, such as determining when a patient can return to work. According to historical literature on work-related mental health issues published by the Royal Australian College of General Practitioners:

GPs are the front line providers of care for growing numbers of patients with work-related mental health conditions. They play a key role in shaping a patient's recovery from point of diagnosis, facilitating access to allied or specialist care and assistance in determining when and how patients can return to work. These guidelines provide evidence to support GPs in managing these patients.[16]

The human resources (HR) sector also plays a key role in workplace health and safety policy and practice, including determining the type of training delivered. Depression and anxiety are at the forefront of many workplace mental health training programs. Furthermore, there is specific, detailed content that further perpetuates Default Depression, such as training workers to:

Recognise the symptoms of the most common types of mental illness, including anxiety, depression and substance abuse

Identify the triggers of depression and suicide[17]

The training organisations delivering workplace mental health training align themselves with, and implicitly endorse, the leadership of the current approach. Beyond Blue was a key pioneer of workplace mental health training in Australia. In their 2004–2005 Annual Report, Beyond Blue describes aspects of its workplace training, and in a glaring example of pathologisation, equates 'symptoms of depression' with 'illness':

Through the program, qualified trainers present professional development sessions to raise awareness of the symptoms of depression, effective treatments and how to approach and assist people with the illness.[18]

The Beyond Blue report details the range of industries and sectors the organisation was already influencing. Since then, Beyond Blue has continued with a deliberate strategy to further its business relationship with the workplace.[19] In many organisations these relationships may have commenced with a genuine goal of ameliorating suffering and assisting human resources staff with difficult and complex issues, but Beyond Blue, with its overt focus on individual mental health, has become so highly influential that industrial relations issues, such as working conditions, have become obscured. Work-related stress is a major cause of occupational ill health, poor productivity and human error;[20] rather than the predominance of a focus on individuals and their mental illness, there are questions about the integrity of the current system. A survey conducted by YouGov online in 2021 found that

One in two (49%) Australian workers feel their workplace has introduced mental health and wellbeing initiatives to 'tick boxes' while day-to-day, their manager shows little if any genuine concern or empathy for their wellbeing [21]

WMH should be seen as an industrial relations issue. Even Black Dog, which generally endorses the medicalised narrative around mental health, believes workplace mental health is an industrial relations issue.[22]

Workplace mental health training is a growing industry with an increasing number of academic papers published on the subject.[23] The growth of Default Depression throughout the corporate sector suits the business interests of well-established organisations that deliver workplace mental health training and facilitated planning sessions. Workplace training in Australia has become a multi-billion-dollar-per-annum business.[24] Much of this is spent on mental health training. The delivery of workplace mental health training programs is now a substantial commercial activity in its own right, both in Australia and internationally. Training providers of WMH often work in business partnerships with high-profile not-for-profit organisations whose own organisational and commercial interests are well-served by the further entrenchment of the current approach with thousands of programs delivered every year; one company alone, the Mental Health Foundation of Australia, delivers 4500 training courses annually.[25]

Safety and workers' wellbeing in the workplace are important workplace responsibilities – the issue is that too often, workplace stress is automatically considered a mental health issue, rather than an issue about the conditions of work.

The stigmatisation of mental health and the social dimension of harm is another workplace issue as it jeopardises employment and promotional opportunities:

Despite the huge drive to raise awareness and challenge this stigma, the workplace remains the environment in which many people feel least comfortable discussing their mental health. A recent UK survey found that despite almost a third (32%) of adults saying they have suffered from mental health problems at work, 49% do not feel there is an appropriate culture in their workplace to enable people to open up about their mental wellbeing. More than half – 54% – said they were not aware what mental health support was available at their workplace. Another UK survey indicated that employers' main concerns were that an employee with a mental health condition would be a threat to safety, incapable of handling stress, demonstrate unpredictable behaviour or underperform. These types of assumptions and negative attitudes must be overcome to foster a truly diverse and inclusive global workforce.[26]

There is good evidence demonstrating similar challenges in Australia with these contradictions that can impact heavily on individual workers. If workers, as they are now being encouraged to do, own up to experiencing distress (regardless of cause or context), they are likely to be encouraged to seek support for this – but as a mental health issue. They will then be directed toward diagnosis of mental disorder, after which they may suffer stigmatisation and employment vulnerability – while the cause of the distress is left unaddressed.

Workplace policies and practices

Support for a stressed worker is often conditional upon the worker accepting the restrictive pathway of a medical appointment where the outcome is most often a diagnosis of depression and the prescription of antidepressants.[27]

This process and pathway are repeated across most workplace contexts: allied health institutions such as palliative care, the media and entertainment, and education at all levels, including the primary school sector, where there has been a significant increase in primary school children being diagnosed with mental disorders including clinical depression, anxiety disorder and attention deficit disorder.[28]

Most Western countries have experienced similar trends in workplace mental health policy and practice, but there is an important difference. In Australia there is a particularly close connection between the insurance industry and the superannuation industry, with well-established business partnerships playing a crucial role in risk-management by insurance companies.[29] The insurance industry often pays out for mental disorder in the workplace as income protection because their superannuation partner has provided this as a part of the worker's superannuation package.[30] For Australian workers, income protection is the principal form of support for extended sick leave, and this covers most Australian wage earners.

Over the last few years in Australia, the financial sector (and in particular the life insurance industry) has become increasingly concerned about the impacts of workplace mental health. A major report from the financial services sector published in 2019 gives a detailed account of substantial increases, including Medicare-subsidised mental health services (increased from 5.7% in 2008/2009 to 9.8% in 2016/2017), and an annual average increase of mental health-related GP encounters of 4.7% since 2011/2012.[31] The report refers to 2016 data from The Australian Institute of Health and Welfare (AIHW), which reveals that in an Australian context, mental illness contributes to 12% of the total burden of disease and 24% of the years lost to disability (the highest proportion of any disease class).[32] The widespread adoption of policies and practices around workplace mental health is a major contributor to the increasing numbers of diagnoses of depression which, in turn, contribute significantly to the escalating diagnoses of mental disorder. Everyone is being hit with escalating costs of this social phenomenon.

In 2019, the *British Medical Journal* published 'Workplace Mental health: a strategic driver of over diagnosis'. It argued:

> *The narrow focus on increasing diagnosis and treatment locates the problem within individuals and deflects attention from the impact of working conditions on mental health and from broader social determinants of mental health. Some WMH [workplace mental health] documents, policies, and programs pay lip-service to these, but nevertheless focus squarely on individualised assessment, diagnosis, and treatment – which in the real world very often means antidepressants and other psychotropic drug treatment.*[33]

Some senior personnel within the Australian financial sector have publicly acknowledged the role of the life insurance industry in the increasing diagnoses for mental health:

> *There was general opinion by key experts that mental health diagnoses are somewhat loosely applied (e.g. self-report of a couple of 'symptoms' can result in a diagnosis). The vast majority of these presenting problems, once labelled 'stress' issues, now attract a disorder diagnosis that leads to potential ineffective 'treatment', i.e. a prescription to manage their 'mood', not address their psychosocial problem/s.*[34]

The Australian federal government reports that the cost of workplace mental ill health in Australia was $12.8 billion in 2015/2016.[35] According to the current figures on the Safe Work Australia website, insurance claims for mental disorder in the workplace now amount to more than $500 million paid in workers' compensation.[36] However, almost 90% of these claims are due to stressful work conditions or events. A Safe Work Australia report, *Work Related Mental Disorders Profile*, published in 2015, is a telling example of the corruption of the experience of distress (see Appendix C).[37] The report highlights 'work-related mental disorders', however it clearly shows that the majority of claims are for issues such as 'Work pressure' – 32%, 'Work related harassment and /or workplace bullying' – 24%, and 'Exposure to workplace or occupational violence' – 15%. Of course, these are all important workplace issues; but they should be addressed as workplace and industrial issues rather than as evidence or symptoms of a clinical mental disorder.

There are important aspects of this trend that need to be changed, including the idea of the provision of clinical treatment for all mental health related workers' compensation claims.[38] Regardless of the factors causing the stress or trauma, in many cases workers on longer term sick leave can only attract payment under income protection once they've been seen by a GP and diagnosed with a mental disorder (usually clinical depression leading to prescription of antidepressants). In Australia, insurance claims involving mental health conditions are typically associated with longer than average time off work and higher than average claim costs.[39]

Institutionalisation and bureaucratisation has become embedded in formal workplace policy and practice. In this context the workplace fulfils its organisational duty-of-care obligations, not by addressing the causes of the stress, but through workplace policy, directing distressed workers toward a medical diagnosis (and often a Mental Health Treatment Plan) to justify the payments for their sick leave. There is an argument to say that this process, of automatically and systematically reducing workers' distress to a mental health issue, replicated across the breadth of organisations in our community, *diminishes* the integrity of individual workers' care.

There are several important dynamics that help maintain the predominance of the current paradigm of illness. Two key examples: general media coverage that supports the profile and general appeal of mental health and the focus on depression, with high-profile media attention given to campaigns such as R U OK?; and government policy and related funding allocations to organisations that benefit financially, but also reputationally, by maintaining their generally accepted leadership profile.[40]

And despite, or perhaps because of, workplace mental health training and substantial funding to mental health awareness programs, 'in many countries the workplace consistently surfaces as the context where people with mental health problems feel stigmatised and discriminated the most'.[41]

Workplace mental health training programs

Training programs are built on ambiguous language, questionable research and misinformation. Training organisations and industry representative bodies build their commercial profile and their training content around key aspects of the current approach, with a focus on depression, including core learning outcomes such as helping workers in 'identifying symptoms of depression', defining depression as an illness and directing people to be diagnosed for a mental illness.

Importantly, some workplace mental health training content modifies (or corrupts) aspects of the World Health Organization (WHO) literature on workplace stress that defines the circumstances and contexts that impact on workers. This language would allow for a less medicalised view of distress; for example, it deliberately and specifically refers to the 'high psychological distress' that can affect workers. However, in Australian workplace mental health training, this language is replaced by terms like 'mental health', 'depression' and 'anxiety', as though they mean the same thing. They often don't.

Signs of distress resulting from workplace stressors are interpreted as the symptoms of a clinical depression. As a result of their training, workers are encouraged, or even mandated, to engage with stressed workers or discreetly with management and human resources about their distressed co-worker.

General misinformation about workplace mental health and the challenges of dealing with worker distress is pervasive within workplace training. It influences many aspects and levels of workplace culture including legal policy and practice in the workplace, for example, legal firms promoting services for employers and employees built around the government's own distorted interpretation of workers compensation claims.

There are a range of types of activities and resources that are offered and these include: one-dimensional programs like brochures on mental health, live yoga webinars, laughter workshops, online mindfulness and movement classes; and the ubiquitous advice to 'talk to someone'. There is nothing wrong with these sorts of activities per se, but they are superficial in the face of the significant challenges of the community or the workplace generally.

This compromised and problematic workplace mental health training is now delivered on a large scale, and across a range of sectors beyond the workplace; in education, where common children's behaviours are diagnosed as mental disorders, and in the employment sector, where many unemployed people are diagnosed as having a medical condition and are moved to a disability pension. Close to 40% of all Disability Support Pension (DSP) recipients (over 300,000 people) have been moved from Newstart (now called JobSeeker), and there is readily available information and guidance to support this process.[42] Legal Aid Victoria, for example, supports unemployed people to apply to Centrelink for the DSP. This step-by-step process includes a template letter for a doctor to ensure the correct medical diagnosis for a clinical mental health condition.[43]

Transition to the DSP from employment follows a similar formalised pathway. The Australian Government's Social Security Guide clearly spells out the guidelines and gives a specific example of how mild depression and anxiety fits with the guidelines for the DSP.[44] This webpage cites the specific Social Security webpage – Mental Health Function – for the assessment of work-related impairment for the Disability Support Pension.[45] Employers have obligations to employees with disabilities, including depression; on behalf of the employer, human resources can follow the federal government's guidelines to advise distressed workers to seek a DSP.[46] The steps, including medical diagnosis for clinical disorders, are clearly set out within this government guidance.

Professional sport is yet another sector that has fully adopted the institutionalised approach to depression. Elite sportspeople with gambling concerns or relationship breakdowns, or who are struggling under media pressure are often referred to, and treated, as having mental health issues, either implied depression or openly described as depression. This approach is not without its critics – a recent article by leading *Age* journalist Greg Baum has critiqued the overemphasis on mental health in sport.[47]

Compounding the challenges of the broader Default Depression context is the lack of effective oversight to ensure quality and up-to-date evidence in training content. For example, there are websites in Australia (even with federal and state government logos) offering training that presents questionable and unsubstantiated information as 'fact'.[48]

The recent response from the life insurance industry to the *Productivity Commission's Draft Report on the Social & Economic Benefits of Improving Mental Health* clearly endorses the need for significant revision of workplace mental health training. The paper recognises that to implement a broadened conceptual approach to worker distress, claims professionals:

> *would require a diverse and well developed skill-set that currently extends beyond current role capabilities. Recruitment strategies and case management practices within life insurers would need to fully consider the skills, knowledge and qualifications necessary to implement a psychosocial model. Multi/interdisciplinary teams for intervention planning need to be coordinated by appropriately qualified and skilled case managers.*
>
> *Case management is a complex role; – mediation and psychosocially focused clinical skills are required.*[49]

A significant challenge for the workplace and the insurance industry is to ensure that language used to describe distress is not strictly clinical, and is appropriately reflected in policy. Throughout workplace mental health literature, terms such as 'mental health', a 'mental health condition' and 'mental health issues' are equated with 'mental illness'.[50] Despite some instances of attempts to use some non-pathologising language, the policies nevertheless strongly tend to direct people toward diagnosis of mental disorder, and the general confusion and ambiguity about definitions and diagnosis from the mental health/ suicide prevention sector is commonly replicated in workplace policy and training programs.[51]

The cost of workplace mental health

As described earlier, the escalating costs for worker compensation and income protection are having a significant impact on the economic viability of the life insurance industry. A major report commissioned by the industry itself describes how this is impacting on consumers' access to cover and compromises the availability of this essential financial support for workers beset with injury or illness.[52] The life insurance industry is a vital financial support mechanism for millions of workers in Australia through income protection and disability income in the case of workplace illness and injury. This financial safety net for workers is commonly available as part of their superannuation package. If this safety net support is lost, the burden will then be shifted onto the government to provide the many millions of dollars necessary to provide this basic support.

> *The sustainability of the life insurance industry, therefore, is a necessary consideration to ensure the financial security of millions of Australians and the sustainability of the social security system.*[53]

In light of this, the life insurance industry has provided a detailed response to the recent federal government's *Productivity Commission's Draft Report on the Social & Economic Benefits of Improving Mental Health*. The response spells out a number of major concerns, including: the large number of mental illness-related claims (now the second-most common cause of claims); the significant losses to the industry by providing income protection insurance cover to members in industries or contexts of elevated risk of mental-illness-related events; and broader challenges in defining what constitutes psychological safety in the workplace and how to measure this.[54]

The life insurance industry is a vital part of our national social support capacity; the industry response report declares that after government, the life insurance industry is the largest financial (and other supports) contributor for people with a mental illness. The significant losses reported by the industry by providing income protection for mental illness are so large that respected leaders in the financial sector are concerned that the current form of the industry itself is not sustainable. The loss of income protection would have a profound effect on our capacity to provide worker support.

The KPMG/FSC report proposes a way forward:

> *Recognising the substantive impact psychosocial domains have on the development and persistence of common mental health problems, as well as other conditions and their associated social, financial and employment impacts, it is clear that strategic change in response to the increasing impact of mental health issues requires reviewing systems and energetic engagement with evidence-based improvements.*

WHO's mental health in the workplace agenda

The World Health Organization (WHO) has taken a strong leadership role in the rise in profile of workplace mental health. However, published concern about the WHO's approach to mental health has come from a broad range of researchers and academics. It covers issues such as: organisational changes that impact work conditions and correlate with increased rates of leave due to 'high [psychological] distress'; the validity of the science involved; and the influence of the pharmaceutical industry.[55]

The WHO plays an important role in perpetuating the ambiguity and confusion around key terms and concepts in the workplace mental health literature. For example, in a recent information sheet, their 'risks to mental health' are clearly of a situational nature, including poor management practice impacting on workers, and bullying and psychosocial harassment. To add to the ambiguity, the WHO explicitly recommends addressing 'mental health problems regardless of cause' – providing an opportunity for the workplace to disregard the cause of the distress.[56]

Workplace stress has attracted major attention on the world stage since at least the early 2000s. According to the WHO, people affected by work stress may suffer a range of symptoms including becoming increasingly distressed and irritable, becoming unable to relax or concentrate and having difficulty sleeping. They may also experience serious physical problems, such as heart disease and increases in blood pressure.[57] Stress can manifest as a range of serious physiological health issues, but this should not be interpreted as symptomatic of mental disorder.

The role of GPs

General practitioners (GPs) have a central role in the institutionalisation of workplace mental health and the Default Depression phenomenon. In Australia, GPs see about 96% of injured workers, and are considered the main gatekeepers to workers' entitlements.[58] For many decades, GPs have played a key role in the challenges of dealing with work-related accidents and injury by providing diagnosis, advice, and facilitating the treatments required for return to work for workplace issues.[59]

The increasing prominence of depression and anxiety as workplace issues is reflected in mental health as a proportion of general practice, and a corresponding challenge for GPs.[60] This burden is likely to increase, with research suggesting the 'symptoms of anxiety and depression' in the workplace are underestimated.[61] We can expect those organisations selling the current approach to WMH to use this to justify continuing to push their business interests (for instance, mental health training) with continued vigour.

For GPs, there are signicant and complex systemic challenges that come with this changing role, in particular the need for better training to equip GPs to manage the complex biopsychosocial factors involved.[62] More specifically, GPs report challenges assessing and diagnosing mental health injuries, and determining the difference between mental illnesses developed *as a result of* work-related stress and those *pre-existing* mental illnesses secondary to work.[63]

In order to move toward more appropriate national and community responses to people in distress, we need to properly address the challenges for GPs, as well as the general medical system, in relation to patients presenting with 'mental health'. We need comprehensive national programs, including appropriate training for workplace mental health for people at all levels of all industry sectors as well as training programs for the whole medical community, including GPs, to ensure there is a wholesale cultural shift in how workplaces navigate this issue.

Chapter 5

Under pressure:
the role of general medical practice

Doctors are at the pointy end of much of the Default Depression process. Escalating numbers of people are being directed to the narrow pathway of a medicalised approach to their distress – and they are coming from every direction and every sector of our community. Schools direct children to GPs for a diagnosis that fits with their organisational policies and obligations; likewise, workplace mental health consultations, sports clubs direct players, friends encourage their friends ...

In Australia, general practitioners (GPs) are therefore often the primary gateway to the mental health system, and for many people, GPs *are* the mental health system; most mental health diagnoses and treatment cases start and finish with the GP.[1] GPs therefore play a pivotal role in Default Depression: of all diagnoses for mental disorder, it is GPs – rather than other medical practitioners, such as psychiatrists – who make the most diagnoses, and they prescribe the most psychiatric drugs.[2] This has brought significant practical, clinical and ethical challenges to the role of GPs and of general medical practice.

Responding to mental health issues has now become the main activity in general practice, with depression being the mental-health-related problem that GPs most frequently manage.[3] GPs prescribe the great majority (86.8%) of all mental health-related prescriptions.[4] The majority of these prescriptions are for antidepressant medications

(67.8%, or 24 million).[5] Following these encounters, however, GPs make referrals at a rate of only 18.8 per 100 mental-health-related problems, and thus continue to manage the vast majority of cases. According to research, the most common management of mental health-related problems was for the GP to prescribe, supply or recommend medication, amounting to 61.6 per 100 cases managed.[6]

GPs are therefore under enormous community, political and corporate pressure to provide some form of mental health treatment to already large – and still increasing – numbers of attending patients. We now have a cultural expectation that GPs, as a part of their day-to-day practice, will routinely diagnose patients in distress for clinical depression and offer treatment that regularly includes prescription antidepressant drugs. The Default Depression culture is so pervasive and firmly established, as evidenced by rigid workplace policy and the continuing well-funded publicity and campaigns around mental health, that many distressed patients presenting to GPs now actually expect this outcome, regardless of the factors involved in their distress. Bureaucracies across industries and other sectors, including education, require a formal diagnosis of mental disorder to provide follow-up support – and there is now a broad expectation that the GP will rubberstamp this process. These challenges have been described in an opinion piece, 'It's rare to be able to tell the truth – here's what's wrong with Australia's mental health system', from a GP working in the Hunter region in NSW, published in the *Guardian* in April 2021.[7]

GPs have long had an integral role in the institutional side of workplace health and safety issues, particularly providing diagnoses and advice, and facilitating the treatments required for returning to work. However, GPs now play an increasingly significant, complex and challenging role in workplace health and safety because of the proliferation of workplace (so-called) mental health issues. For large numbers of distressed workers who visit their GP, once they are diagnosed with a mental disorder such as clinical depression or anxiety disorder and have satisfied workplace requirements around this process, they are unlikely to have contact with other aspects of the mental health system. Nevertheless, their experience with a GP has them listed as having engaged with the *mental health system*, significantly skewing the figures for 'engagement with the mental health system'.

General challenges for GPs

GPs face many challenges when providing appropriate professional support to people in distress.[8] According to their own representative organisations, GPs are overworked, with many GPs reporting that their excessive workloads can prevent them from providing high-quality care.[9] GPs have limited referral options, so people in distress that need support for issues that might be addressed outside the health system – such as highly stressful financial or legal difficulties – are generally left wanting. Further compounding the challenges to providing appropriate support, and regardless of the good intentions of GPs, treatment outcomes for depression are significantly impacted by the adverse social contexts of patients.[10]

Many GPs are concerned about over diagnosis, and the medicalising of common human distress and the serious harm that can come from this. Leading international primary health care academics Christopher Dowrick, UK professor of primary medical care, and Allen Frances, US emeritus professor of psychiatry, have stated that depression is 'now more likely to be over diagnosed than under diagnosed in primary care'.[11] A key factor in over diagnosis, as GPs themselves see it, is the inadequate criteria for diagnosing mental disorders, especially depression. As we have seen, the criteria for depression are broad and lack precision:

> The criteria, which have not changed since 1980, capture too heterogeneous a population for research studies and are so loose that, in everyday clinical practice, ordinary sadness can be easily confused with clinical depression.[12]

Simply put, grief and anxiety can be interpreted as the symptoms of a clinical depression, leading to an understandable over diagnosis of depression and, in so doing, inflation of the perceived prevalence of mental disorders.

Further compounding the difficulties for GPs around clinical diagnosis is that the scientific validity of *Diagnostic and Statistical Manual of Mental Disorders* (DSM) on which GP screening tools and clinical guidelines are often based, has long been questioned.[13] Dowrick and Frances are among those who have expressed concern about how the poor diagnostic criteria create serious challenges for everyday clinical practice and are quite forthright about this: 'the approach to diagnosis and management of depression should change'.[14] Scientific validity issues aside, the fact is, in practice, some GPs recognise that important parameters, established by the writers of the DSM series, which are supposedly designed to ensure quality diagnosis, have historically been 'generally ignored'.[15]

The prevalence and complexity of patients experiencing psychological or emotional distress create an especially onerous and highly stressful workload for GPs. Compounding the difficulties of day-to-day general practice are the lack of resources and arduous patient management issues for those presenting with high-intensity mental health challenges, such as schizophrenia, psychosis and personality disorders. Put plainly, many GPs see dealing with mental disorders as 'burdensome'.[16] And from a broader perspective, with the ever-growing profile of mental health and greater numbers of people being directed to general practice for mental health concerns, GPs are concerned about the overall future of mental health.[17]

While the fierce scientific debates about the efficacy and harm of antidepressant drugs continue, overworked and under-resourced GPs are left to navigate the pressure and day-to-day challenges of 'depression treatment options'.[18] GPs and psychiatrists have very different views about what depression is and how to treat it.[19] Research published in the *International Journal of Qualitative Studies on Health and Well-Being* in 2014 suggests that the background clinical context of diagnosis and treatment for depression is itself problematic. While the diagnosis of depression and the guidelines for treatment of patients is developed by psychiatrists, most patients with depression are treated exclusively by GPs. According to this research, GPs and psychiatrists differed considerably in their opinion about the usefulness of the concept of depression. Psychiatrists considered the diagnosis of depression as a pragmatic and agreed construct and they did not question its validity. GPs, on the other hand, thought depression was a 'gray area' and questioned its clinical utility in general practice. GPs in the study were also sceptical about instruments used for measuring depression and felt they could be misleading.

GPs must consider the appropriate treatment response for someone presenting with 'symptoms of depression', including those patients expecting the prescribing of antidepressants – even if a GP is uncertain about this as a treatment option.

On a simple, practical level, GPs are generally time poor and treating psychological or emotional distress is complex and time consuming. Time constraints are one of the key limitations to GPs' capacity to provide quality care.[20]

GPs have rarely undertaken the necessary training to deal effectively with psychological or emotional distress, while general practice organisations themselves consider GPs as often under-trained to meet the demands of those suffering psychological or emotional distress, or mental health disorders.[21]

Ethical challenges in diagnosing depression and anxiety

There are significant ethical challenges for GPs in dealing with patients suffering psychological or emotional distress, including those related to confidentiality, especially within the workplace context. A diagnosis of a mental disorder for a patient following up on a workplace mental health issue will usually be related back to the human resources department of that workplace, at the very least, as the fulfilment of the conditions for ongoing workplace support for the distressed worker. Accordingly, overt changes will be made at the workplace to accommodate this, potentially compromising the confidentiality.

Other ethical challenges for GPs relate to the prescription of antidepressants, the efficacy of which is challenged by strong evidence questioning fundamental aspects of previous research that indicated positive outcomes with antidepressants.[22]

In many cases, antidepressants are prescribed as first-line treatment, contrary to explicit recommendations from peak bodies, like this position statement from the Royal College of Psychiatrists in the UK:

> *Antidepressant use among children and adolescents should only be part of second-line treatment for moderate to severe depression when patients are unresponsive to psychological therapy.*[23]

The prescribing of antidepressants, whether or not they are recommended as first-line treatment, may cause serious harm. Mainstream media has reported the horrific effects of antidepressants on primary school-age children – 'Children prescribed anti-depressants for anxiety that "made them suicidal" and 'Aged just seven, my girl became death-obsessed'.[24] While some of these reports are about individual instances only, they are powerful and valid accounts of horrendous ordeals; and they add to the argument for the need for a more open and thorough review of this topic.

When prescribing antidepressants, GPs must weigh up the potential treatment support versus the potential serious side effects,[25] including:

- the increased risk of suicide and violence at all ages[26]
- anxiety, agitation, panic attacks, insomnia, irritability, hostility, aggressiveness, impulsivity, akathisia (psychomotor restlessness), hypomania, and mania[27]
- withdrawal difficulties that can be dangerous. There are severe and persistent withdrawal reactions that affect up to 50% of antidepressant users, and there are other severe physical dependence issues. Withdrawal from antidepressants often requires considerable time and care and ongoing monitoring of withdrawal symptoms.[28]

These side effects, and potential harms from the use of antidepressants, are explored in more depth in the next chapter.

Chapter 6

Medicating human distress: effectiveness and harms from antidepressants

When we systematically interpret and diagnose common human experience as mental disorder – often as clinical depression – and then we medicate with potentially harmful drugs, commonly antidepressants, we medicalise distress. Martin Whitely describes this process pointedly:

> *At the heart of the problem is how we have come to define mental health and mental illness. Anything that causes us to be sad, stressed, anxious, or even bored is now regarded as a threat to our mental health, and therefore a potential source of mental illness. If you lose your job, are grieving a death or a relationship breakdown, or are experiencing any of life's inevitable vicissitudes, then it is very human to be deeply unhappy or anxious and some may even fleetingly consider ending it all. But we have come to regard these normal, although troubling, human reactions as compelling evidence of mental illness.[1]*

We have created a cultural and institutional phenomenon around the clinical category of depression – and we prescribe antidepressants to treat the depression. However, the history, science and culture of clinical depression, and the use of antidepressants, has been plagued by contradictory research. Are, in fact, antidepressants an effective treatment for clinical depression? And what are the potential harms? There are major concerns about harmful, addictive and/or dependence impacts and issues across the whole population,[2] including increased suicidality from antidepressants among children, as well as the challenges and potentially harmful outcomes from withdrawal from antidepressants.[3]

Rising antidepressant prescription rates

During the last several decades, diagnoses of clinical depression and anxiety disorder have risen, with a consequential massive increase in the numbers and rates of prescribed antidepressants across much of the globe.[4] A 2017 report from the Organisation for Economic Co-operation and Development (OECD) showed that the consumption of antidepressant drugs doubled in OECD countries between 2000 and 2015.[5] An article in *Business Insider* revealed that in Germany, antidepressant use had risen 46% in just four years. In Spain and Portugal, antidepressant use rose about 20% during the same period.[6] There have been substantial increases in many countries on most continents; this is a worldwide trend.

In the United States, antidepressant use has increased by nearly 65% over 15 years, from 7.7% in 1999–2002, to 12.7% in 2011–2014.[7] The US, which is not included in the OECD data, has the highest rate of antidepressant use in the world.[8]

Prescriptions for antidepressants in England have almost doubled in number in the past decade, with 2018 recording a record number.[9]

According to OECD reports, Australia is now listed as having one of the highest rates of antidepressant drug consumption.[10] Antidepressants are taken by around 10% of adult Australians each day, making it the most commonly used medication in Australia.[11]

In 2020–2021, 4.5 million patients (17.7% of the Australian population) filled a prescription for a mental health-related medication, with an average of 9.4 prescriptions per patient. Of these, 73.1% were for antidepressant medications, and a total of 42.7 million mental health-related medications (subsidised and under co-payment) were dispensed. The vast majority, 84.7%, were prescribed by GPs, with 7.5% prescribed by psychiatrists and 4.9% by non-psychiatrist specialists.

During 2019–2020, the Australian Government spent $566 million, or $22 per Australian, on subsidised mental health-related prescriptions under the PBS/RPBS. Prescriptions for antipsychotics (48.1%) and antidepressants (32.5%) accounted for the majority of this, followed by prescriptions for psychostimulants, agents used for attention deficit hyperactivity disorder (ADHD) and nootropics (13.1%), anxiolytics (4.1%), and hypnotics and sedatives (2.2%).[12]

In the six years to 2019–2020, the number of children aged 17 years of age and under on antidepressant medication in Australia increased to 115,482 – a 62.7% increase from 2013–2014. This includes 628 children aged 0–4 years.[13]

The extent of this overprescribing impacts on people of all ages, including those in the aged-care sector. A recent study, submitted to the Royal Commission into Aged Care Quality and Safety, found that:

Nearly two-thirds (61%) [of 11,368 residents] were taking psycho-tropic agents regularly, with over 41% prescribed antidepressants, 22% antipsychotics and 22% of residents taking benzodiazepines … More than 16% of the residents were taking sedating antidepressants, predominantly mirtazapine.[14]

The concerns about inappropriate drug use in aged care include the widespread single or combined use of antidepressants in older adults and the increase in serotonin syndrome[15] and the marked increase in older people receiving psychotropic medicines after they enter residential care.[16]

Effectiveness of antidepressants

The science around the effectiveness of antidepressants is plagued with controversy and contradictory research. Some research suggests antidepressants can be effective in treating depression, and advocates for the use of antidepressants, such as organisations representing medical practitioners, refer to this research when developing guidelines for the use of drugs as treatment. However, for all the research that supports the use of antidepressants, there is a good deal of peer-reviewed evidence that represents a case for serious caution, at the very least, in regard to their use.

The growing inexactitude and confusion around antidepressant research compounds the challenges for general medical practice. There is no reliable evidence on who benefits most from which treatment, and variable responses means treatment plans and drugs should be tailored based on more detailed patient background information – information that may not be readily available to a GP.[17]

Recent research articles by Irving Kirsch, Wojciech Oronowicz-Jaśkowiak and Przemysław Bąbel, and Michael Hengartner and Martin Plöderl highlight the important role that the placebo effect plays in clinical trials.[18] For example:

> *analyses of the published and the unpublished clinical trial data are consistent in showing that most (if not all) of the benefits of antidepressants in the treatment of depression and anxiety are due to the placebo response, and the difference in improvement between drug and placebo is not clinically meaningful.*

This accords with earlier research.[19]

The theory of an association between serotonin and depression has been soundly rejected. A 2022 review of the evidence found that while the serotonin hypothesis of depression is still influential,

> *The main areas of serotonin research provide no consistent evidence of there being an association between serotonin and depression, and no support for the hypothesis that depression is caused by lowered serotonin activity or concentration.*[20]

Others assert that there has been selectivity in the publication of research into antidepressants with a bias toward the publication of positive results.[21]

While there will always be debate about appropriate research methodology and interpretation of results, the potential harms of antidepressants are broadly and openly acknowledged.

Harms from antidepressants

As shown earlier, in Australia we have one of the highest rates of antidepressant use among OECD countries with a growth rate that continues.[22] The dramatic increase in the rates of diagnosis of clinical depression and prescribing of antidepressants drugs over the last few decades has happened despite considerable numbers of books, peer-reviewed research articles and other papers and reports spelling out the potential harms from these drugs.[23] The prescribing of antidepressants for children is particularly concerning. A major review by Australian Child Psychiatrist Professor Jon Jureidini, published in the *Lancet*, describes how antidepressants are ineffective and harmful for children and adolescents.[24] The *Sydney Morning Herald* published an article about the *Lancet* paper:

> *Antidepressants prescribed for children are ineffective and may cause serious harm, including suicide attempts, a major review shows.*
>
> *The findings had 'disturbing implications' for treating major depression in children, ... as the use of antidepressants and antipsychotics continues to rise among children as young as two years old. ... the rate of serious harms linked to other antidepressants, including paroxetine, sertraline, and citalopram may be underestimated due to selective reporting, the burying of unpublished trials showing adverse effects and poorly designed trials.[25]*

As part of their product labelling, the US Federal Drug Administration offers quite a list of symptoms associated with the use of antidepressants:

> *The following symptoms, anxiety, agitation, panic attacks, insomnia, irritability, hostility, aggressiveness, impulsivity, akathisia (psychomotor restlessness), hypomania, and mania, have been reported in adult and pediatric patients being treated with*

*antidepressants for major depressive disorder as well as for other
indications, both psychiatric and nonpsychiatric.*[26]

The harms from antidepressants include increased risk of
suicidality, other dangerous side effects listed below, problematic
withdrawal, and the potential for addiction and stigmatisation.
Antidepressants are also used for intentional over-dosing.[27] Research
published in 2020 asserts that there are also associations between
maternal antidepressant use and specific birth defects.[28]

The selective use, or cherry picking, of results from the breadth of
research that is available is common. It is used to bolster the messaging
of the business interests of research institutions, training organisations
and other not-for-profits, and it supports the continuing predominance
of the medicalised mental health paradigm and the Default Depression
response to distress.

This is not to say, however, that there is no case for the use of
antidepressants; rather, the concern is that too often antidepressants
are prescribed as a default response to any number of behaviours and
responses associated with stressful situations.

Antidepressants increase the risk of suicide and death at all ages

Antidepressants increase the suicide risk in children and adolescents.[29]
It is concerning, therefore, to think that in Australia, despite this
clear warning, schools are encouraged to develop policies around
mental illness, without due consideration for the context of the child's
behaviour or distress.[30] This trend, part of a strong push to further
medicalise children's behaviour, currently focuses on anxiety, but
the persuasive push toward diagnoses of depression and attention
deficit disorders is still common.[31] The consequence is that it justifies
the prescribing of harsh antidepressant and antipsychotic drugs to
children.

That antidepressants increase suicidality in children and adolescents has been accepted for almost two decades, and it is acknowledged
by the US Federal Drug Administration (FDA), which requires

information on drug packaging to spell this out.[32] More recently, research has shown that antidepressants significantly increase the suicide risk in adults.[33]

There is also evidence that antidepressants increase the risk of violence, increase the risk of death in the general population, and increase the risk of death in certain health conditions.[34]

Antidepressants, aggression and violence

There is sound evidence supporting the association of antidepressants with violence and aggression. The *British Medical Journal* (*BMJ*) published an article in 2017 that stated:

There is enough creditable evidence supporting the association of antidepressants with violence and aggression to warrant comprehensive, open investigation and research to properly understand this important issue.[35]

This evidence includes published research and well-constructed media articles revealing an association between antidepressants and violence and aggression, including murder. While there is still debate and uncertainty about causality, it has been conceded that some level of causality does exist. David Healy pointed out in the *BMJ* in 2017:

Causality has been conceded by prosecutors, regulators, and companies. As early as 1983, Pfizer noted that antidepressants could cause aggressive behaviour.[36]

Antidepressants have been implicated in murders, and used as a defence in a number of murder trials. This includes several successful cases where the defence of using antidepressants has led to a reduced sentence or even acquittal where juries have accepted that the defendants' behaviour and personality had been changed dramatically due to the prescribed antidepressant medications.

A newspaper report in 2017 referred to a BBC investigation that described how 'Using Freedom of Information laws, BBC *Panorama* found 28 cases where the drugs have been implicated in a murder'. The report stated:

Citizens Commission on Human Rights (CCHR) International, a mental health watchdog that has been documenting the effects of psychotropic drugs for 48 years, especially violent and suicidal effects, said the documentary vindicates many experts and advocacy groups that have warned about such dangers. The group says it should serve as a catalyst for law enforcement officers, coroners, and the courts to investigate psychotropic drug links to acts of violence.[37]

A thorough investigation of dozens of perpetrators of mass killings by the CCHR has described how many were either on antidepressants at the time of their rampage, had abruptly quit taking their medication when they went on their spree, or had been prescribed antidepressants at some point in the past.[38]

The side effects from antidepressants are openly acknowledged

The FDA warns about the many side effects of antidepressants listed earlier. Severe and persistent withdrawal reactions affect up to 50% of antidepressant users, and there are other severe physical dependence issues.[39] And it is not only the FDA who offers these warnings. Other important respected institutions, including the Royal College of Psychiatrists in the UK and the National Health System (NHS) in the UK, also openly report the harmful side effects of these drugs.[40] The NHS's list of side effects includes: sexual dysfunction, premature delivery for pregnant women and delivering babies of lower birth weight, as well as dangers from reactions with other drugs.

Despite the clear warnings about the dangers of antidepressants and other similar drugs, they are prescribed in large numbers to children. Martin Whitely studied the *Therapeutic Goods Administration's Public Case Detail* reports, which listed children's reactions to such drugs. Whitely describes a sample from the Adverse Drug Reactions Committee (ADRAC) adverse event reports for atomoxetine hydrochloride (Strattera). Straterra was originally trialled as an antidepressant but is now used as a drug for ADHD.[41] Whitely presented the following list of reactions by children to Straterra:

- *8-year-old boy who 'hit his head against a wall' and had 'thoughts of suicide – stating that he wants to kill himself'*
- *12-year-old girl who experienced 'anorexia, weight loss, fidgeting and compulsive behaviour that included ripping out fingernails and toenails, picking and cutting clothing, and anger outbursts'*
- *9-year-old boy who slammed 'his head against walls, had extreme mood swings, violent outbursts' and was 'always angry, depressed or sad and said he wanted to kill himself'*
- *7-year-old girl who experienced 'abdominal pain, nausea, severe right-sided headache, shooting pains, white spots in visual fields, academic regression and faecal and urinary incontinence'*
- *7-year-old boy who experienced 'suicidal ideation and mood changes' and suffered from 'increased aggression' and 'threats to self with knife, picking his skin, poking self with knife'.*[42]

As already stated, there are now over 100,000 children in Australia who have been prescribed antidepressants, with many suffering side effects from common antidepressants, like those listed above. This is despite the fact that no antidepressant is approved by the Therapeutic Goods Administration (TGA) for the treatment of depression or anxiety in Australians aged under 18 years. There are numerous anecdotal accounts of the harm, including from parents whose children are severely traumatised and suicidal.[43] The mounting evidence of the harm for children and adolescents from antidepressants has triggered the Federal Health Minister, Mark Butler MP, to order the development of new evidence-based guidelines for their safe use.[44]

Withdrawal from antidepressants can be highly problematic
Severe and persistent withdrawal reactions affect up to 50% of antidepressant users.[45] This is not an incidental issue. Withdrawal from antidepressants can be dangerous and requires considerable time and care, with ongoing monitoring of withdrawal symptoms.[46]

New research into antidepressant withdrawal and the need to

improve patient safety are described in medical editor Melissa Davey's *Guardian* article, 'Urgent need to find safe ways to withdraw from antidepressants'.[47] One of the key research findings is that studies in this field do not distinguish between symptoms of a return or relapse of depression, and symptoms of withdrawal after stopping antidepressant use.[48] As mentioned earlier, symptoms suffered during withdrawal are sometimes misdiagnosed as symptoms of other disorders. The response is to sometimes prescribe further drug treatments, compounding the patient's suffering.[49] The Royal College of Psychiatrists in the UK has updated its guidelines on withdrawal from antidepressants. The list of 'Symptoms of antidepressant withdrawal' is more than a little sobering:

- *dizziness (this is usually mild, but can be so bad that you can't stand up without help)*
- *anxiety which comes and goes, sometimes in intense 'surges'*
- *difficulty in getting to sleep and vivid or frightening dreams*
- *low mood, feeling unable to be interested in or enjoy things*
- *a sense of being physically unwell*
- *rapidly changing moods*
- *anger, sleeplessness, tiredness, loss of co-ordination and headache*
- *the feeling of an electric shock in your arms, legs, or head (those are sometimes called 'zaps' and turning your head to the side can make them worse)*
- *a feeling that things are not real ('derealisation'), or a feeling that you have 'cotton wool in your head'*
- *difficulty in concentrating*
- *suicidal thoughts*
- *queasiness*
- *a feeling of inner restlessness and inability to stay still (akathisia).*

The Royal College of Psychiatrists' guidelines also openly acknowledge that 'the causes of antidepressant withdrawal symptoms [are] still poorly understood'. And that:

Between a third and half of people who take an antidepressant will experience such symptoms to some extent. We cannot yet predict who will get these symptoms.

The risk seems to be greater if you have taken a high dose for a long time, but it can happen if you have taken an antidepressant for just a month. It can also depend on the type of antidepressant you have been taking. You are more likely to get these symptoms (and for them to be worse) if you stop taking an antidepressant suddenly or if you reduce the dose quickly.[50]

The article in the *Guardian* describes both these guidelines from the Royal College of Psychiatrists in the UK, and the information provided by the Royal Australian and New Zealand College of Psychiatrists (RANZCP) about this topic, as 'vague'.[51] Indeed, much of the information on antidepressants in the RANZCP 'Mood Disorders' article is surprisingly imprecise.[52]

Perhaps of even greater concern, in the information it provides about safety and side effects, the RANZCP in fact recommends prescribing other potentially harmful drugs to counter the side effects of the prescribed antidepressants:

The activation/agitation observed with the initial stages of taking an SSRI can be managed with a low dose of a benzodiazepine prescribed for a limited period of time.[53]

Along with challenges of withdrawal, there is evidence of the misuse and abuse of antidepressants, including psychological dependence and addiction issues.[54]

The pharmaceutical industry prevails despite major legal challenges

Despite all the creditable evidence demonstrating the harms from antidepressants, the extraordinary trend of prescribing these potentially harmful drugs continues, a trend influenced by the success of pharmaceutical companies in suppressing adverse information. Not only have pharmaceutical companies shaped fundamental aspects of the culture around depression and anxiety through investment in research and the development of clinical guidelines, but also their financial magnitude has enabled them to influence the legal and justice systems.[55]

There has been a history of lawsuits, investigation of fraud and substantial out-of-court settlements with the major sellers of antidepressants and antipsychotics, as detailed by Harriet Fraad:

All 30 of the available antidepressants have suffered lawsuits within five years of their appearance on the market. These suits are often settled with large payments and gag clauses. The new generation of anti-psychotics are the latest case in point. Anti-psychotics were the single biggest targets of the False Claims Act. *Every major company selling anti-psychotics – Bristol Meyers Squibb, Eli Lilly, Pfizer, Johnson and Johnson and AstraZeneca – has either settled investigations for healthcare fraud or is currently being investigated for it. Two recent settlements involving charges of illegal marketing set records for the largest criminal fines ever imposed on corporations. Their corporate logic is expressed in the words of Dr Jerome Avorn, a medical professor and researcher at Harvard: 'When you are selling a billion a year or more of a drug, it's very tempting for a company to just ignore the traffic ticket and keep speeding.*[56]

A number of these lawsuits result in fines and settlement costs amounting to hundreds of millions of dollars, with several cases amounting to more than a billion dollars.[57]

It is perplexing to see how deeply Default Depression has become embedded in our society, despite the strong evidence outlining the harms often associated with these drugs. And it is disturbing to see, despite this evidence, how strongly the accepted leaders of the mental health/suicide prevention sector continue to push this approach.

Chapter 7

The role of the pharmaceutical industry

The pharmaceutical industry has played a key role in promoting the interrelated ideas of a clinical depression as a category of mental disorder, and of the use of antidepressants to treat this disorder. Along with the research referenced in this book, there has been a great deal of published material on this topic, including a number of key books and papers by Robert Whitaker, Peter Breggin, Peter C. Gotzsche and Australia's Martin Whitely and Melissa Raven.[1]

The very idea of clinical depression being regarded as a specific clinical condition continues to be clouded with controversy, and contradictory and changing definitions, even within the medical psychiatric community.[2] Despite these fundamental concerns around the definition of mental disorders and the efficacy of prescription drugs, the marketing of antidepressant and antipsychotic drugs by large multinational pharmaceutical companies has continued unabated across the globe.

Sales for antidepressants are among the highest sales of pharmaceuticals in the world

Selling antidepressant drugs is a huge global business. Martin Whitely has written specifically on this theme:

> *And Big Pharma, the senior partner, is not just big, it is huge and getting bigger, with very healthy profit margins. The pharmaceutical*

industry's total global revenue in 2018 was over US$1.2 trillion (US$1,200,000,000,000 – about the size of Australia's GDP) and has grown rapidly from US$390 billion in 2001.[3]

Drug companies generally, including those with significant business in a range of antidepressants and antipsychotics, have spent, and continue to spend, huge amounts of money on marketing. Pharmaceutical advertising topped US$6.58 billion in the US alone in 2020.[4] The global antidepressant market was worth US$11.67 billion in 2019, and retail sales for some individual drugs, including leading brand antidepressants, are in the billions of dollars.[5] The global antidepressant market is projected to reach US$18.29 billion by 2027.[6]

Pharmaceutical companies' marketing budgets have increased from US$17.7 billion to US$29.9 billion from 1997 to 2016. In fact, *pharmaceutical companies spend more on advertising and promotion than on research and development.*[7] It is no wonder that this exerts substantial power and influence in health and mental health sectors across the globe.

The pharmaceutical industry exerts political and financial influence throughout the medical sector

The pharmaceutical industry wields substantial global political and economic influence. In his PhD, Martin Whitely writes of 'overwhelming evidence of regulatory capture by pharmaceutical companies of government drug approval and subsidisation processes that reinforces the dominance of pseudo-scientific Biological Psychiatry'.[8] A recent article in *Frontiers in Research Metrics and Analytics* offers a scathing description of how pharmaceutical companies influence medical science:

There is now abundant evidence that the involvement of pharmaceutical companies corrupts medical science. Within the medical community, this is generally assumed to be the result of conflicts of interest. However, some important ways that the industry corrupts are not captured well by standard analyses in terms of conflicts of interest. It is not just that there is a body of medical science perverted by industry largesse. Instead, much of the corruption of medical science via the pharmaceutical industry happens through grafting activities: Pharmaceutical companies do their own research and smoothly integrate it with medical science, taking advantage of the legitimacy of the latter.[9]

In 2022, the *BMJ* published an article entitled 'The Illusion of evidence-based medicine' by Professor Jon Jureidini. In it he describes how the data from medical research and the ideal of evidence-based medicine is compromised by the pharmaceutical industry.

The advent of evidence-based medicine was a paradigm shift intended to provide a solid scientific foundation for medicine. The validity of this new paradigm, however, depends on reliable data from clinical trials, most of which are conducted by the pharmaceutical industry and reported in the names of senior academics. The release into the public domain of previously confidential pharmaceutical industry documents has given the medical community valuable insight into the degree to which industry-sponsored clinical trials are misrepresented.

Until this problem is corrected, evidence-based medicine will remain an illusion.[10]

Jureidini continues with some detail about how the corruption happens:

Scientific progress is thwarted by the ownership of data and knowledge because industry suppresses negative trial results, fails to report adverse events, and does not share raw data with the academic research community. Patients die because of the adverse impact of commercial interests on the research agenda, universities, and regulators.

Pharmaceutical companies sponsor medical mental health seminars and training programs for GPs and allied health professionals, and provide literature to general practice and for general distribution.[11] They also sponsor and partner with not-for-profit mental health organisations; a 2006 *Age* article linked the Mental Health Council of Australia 'directly to global pharmaceutical giants Pfizer, Eli Lilly, Glaxo SmithKline, Bristol Myers Squibb, Lundbeck, Wyeth and AstraZeneca'.[12] Pharmaceutical companies have been integrally involved in the development of clinical practice guidelines and they have funded the development of depression screening tools – the very tools that are used to determine that a person has a clinical depression.[13] Other research shows how the changing definitions of mental disorders have suited the phenomenal growth in marketing specific types of antidepressants since the late 1980s.[14]

Pharmaceutical companies have been instrumental in the medicalisation of normal behaviour as a part of their marketing strategy. They have created specific new 'disorders' to suit the marketing of specific drugs. Conrad and Slodden, in the *Handbook of the Sociology of Mental Health* describe several examples of this, including discussion about

> *the emergence of social anxiety disorder (SAD) as a common diagnosis, focusing on how a pharmaceutical company initially marketed shyness and social anxiety as a disorder and then advertised Paxil as its preferred treatment.*[15]

Reputable journals have published papers demonstrating the close connection between the pharmaceutical companies and the culture and thinking around depression:

> *drug marketing portrays idealized scientific relationships between psychopharmaceuticals and depression; how multiple stakeholders, including scientists, regulatory agencies, and patient advocacy groups, negotiate neurobiological explanations of mental illness; and how the placebo effect has become a critical issue in these debates, including the possible role of drug advertising to influence the placebo effect directly. We argue that if and how antidepressants*

'work' is not a straightforward objective question, but rather a larger social contest involving scientific debate, the political history of the pharmaceutical industry, cultural discourses surrounding the role of drugs in society, and the interpretive flexibility of personal experience.[16]

This pathologisation, as it relates to depression and the nexus with the development and marketing of antidepressants, has been well described:

A major consequence of the DSM-III's new categorizations was to make depression a more promising target for the new class of antidepressants – the selective serotonin reuptake inhibitors (SSRIs) – that came on the market in the late 1980s. The SSRIs now dominate the treatment of nonpsychotic mental disorders, including MDD and the various anxiety disorders as well as many other conditions. In practice, there is little evidence that the SSRIs' efficacy has any relationship to the diagnostic categories in the DSM. They act very generally to increase levels of serotonin in the brain that both raise low mood states and lower levels of anxiety, so when they first appeared in the late 1980s, the antidepressant SSRIs could just as easily have been marketed as antianxiety medications.[17]

Crucially, pharmaceutical companies market directly to doctors, in various ways, including via GP training programs and other medical education events. An Australian study, published in the *BMJ* in 2016, investigated the relationship between industry-sponsored education events for the medical profession and the over diagnosis and over treatment of several conditions including depression. The paper found that 'primary care clinicians were often targeted, dinner was often provided and that a few companies sponsored most events'.[18]

It is argued that this process influences physician-prescribing rates. 'Interactions between physicians and the pharmaceutical industry', a research paper published in the *BMJ* in 2017, concluded that:

Physician–pharmaceutical industry and its sales representative's interactions and acceptance of gifts from the company's PSRs [pharmaceutical sales representative] have been found to affect physicians' prescribing behaviour and are likely to contribute to irrational prescribing of the company's drug.[19]

The money spent by big pharma on this sector is not wasted; it is used strategically. Published research shows that some prescriptions issued by physicians have been in response to sales representatives deliberately targeting doctors, including by the giving of gifts.[20]

The pharmaceutical companies influence opinion leaders in the medical sector.[21] And they have financial relationships with the organisations that produce clinical practice guidelines[22] – although this is sometimes done covertly. Research into the relationship between the authors of clinical practice guidelines and the pharmaceutical industry in 2016 concluded that:

Financial relationships between organizations that produce clinical practice guidelines and biomedical companies are common and infrequently disclosed in guidelines. Our study highlights the need for an effective policy to manage organizational conflicts of interest and disclosure of financial relationships.[23]

The same conclusion has been drawn by others.[24]

In Australia, the pharmaceutical industry also engages large numbers of paid lobbyists and donates heavily to both major political parties, significantly influencing the development of policy and practice in the medical sector.[25] Pharmaceutical companies also sponsor key not-for-profit organisations in the mental health sector, including leading advocacy groups.[26]

Pharmaceutical companies continue to develop their marketing techniques and reach. A paper published in 2022 in the *Journal of Medical Internet Research* investigates direct-to-consumer marketing. The article describes how pharmaceutical companies:

have found ways to build relationships directly with patients using covert persuasion tactics like partnering with social media influencers.[27]

The pharmaceutical industry has therefore been a major contributor to the growth of the Default Depression approach to distress. In turn, it has benefited and profited enormously from the focus on depression by the leadership of mental health/suicide prevention sector. These political and economic dynamics have been instrumental in establishing and maintaining the pervasive – and largely ineffective – beliefs and practices of the current approaches to mental health and suicide prevention.

Chapter 8

The language of mental health and the illness paradigm

The use of specific language and terminology within the general mental health context and the mental health/suicide prevention sector serves to perpetuate the biomedical response to distress and other common human behaviours. The current approach is rife with ambiguity and misinformation. And within this, the key terms 'depression' and 'anxiety' are used in highly ambiguous ways.

The ambiguity of the term 'depression' complicates and undermines the consideration of appropriate and effective support – whether clinical or social – for people in psychological or emotional distress.

Using language of a clinical or technical nature helps preserve the idea that the provision of support for people in distress should be largely limited to clinicians such as GPs and psychiatrists. For example, using screening tools to determine clinical depression suggests a highly specialised process, when, in fact, most screening tools are little more than a checklist of common behaviours and feelings, described as 'symptoms'.

The language that is used can shape someone's life.

To describe common feelings and behaviours – like depressed mood, loss of confidence or self-esteem, or the diminished ability to concentrate, think or make decisions – as *symptoms* is already shaping the way appropriate support is considered. Use of specific, particularly technical, language – like 'diagnostic tools', 'depression assessment instruments' and 'depression rating scales' – is a key part of the process of medicalisation. Likewise, this approach places important, diverse aspects of people's lives in the hands of clinical medical practitioners (especially doctors and psychiatrists) where in some cases at least, other professional support – for example, vocational support for someone who is unemployed – may be more appropriate. Deferring to screening tools and treatment pathways that respond to common human behaviours in these pathologising, restrictive ways has lifelong implications. It can mean that a person can be diagnosed as having a clinical depression – and therefore, and maybe forever after, labelled as someone with a mental illness – for having merely ticked a relatively small number of boxes that describe common human behaviours and feelings.

However, as we have seen, there is no discrete, scientifically verifiable pathogenic biological or neurological state or condition for depression. Instead, clinical diagnosis is generally based on a sum score of symptoms that are, in fact, common but imprecise emotional or psychological experiences or states.[1] The literature and the general use of the terms 'depression', 'anxiety' and 'mental health' are rife with ambiguity and contradiction; consequently, it can be argued that much of the research and measuring tools for depression and anxiety may be invalid and, further, that clinical practice based on this research may well be unsound. And yet both public and private health and mental health sectors continue to use this ambiguous terminology in developing policy and planned activity. This culture spreads throughout society, as all other sectors plan their mental health activity based on the leadership of the current approach.

This issue is not simply a matter of semantics or somewhat imprecise definitions; the harm resulting from inappropriate diagnosis of depression and other mental 'disorders', and the prescribing of potentially harmful antidepressant and antipsychotic drugs, is already at an alarming level, and is likely to keep rising. As discussed in previous chapters, this is a result of the deliberate, strategic marketing and messaging of the key players of the current approach, including the pharmaceutical industry and high-profile not-for-profit organisations that continue to promote the biomedical approach to distress.

The mental health narrative is built on ambiguity, confusion and misinformation

The broadscale ambiguity of the Default Depression culture suits the operation of leading agencies of the current approach – they can continue to offer superficial descriptions and recommendations for dealing with, or treating, 'depression', but take no responsibility for any unsatisfactory outcomes of their recommendations.

A key factor in the ambiguity is that meanings – including clinical definitions – have changed over the last few decades,[2] and it can be argued that this has suited the marketing of antidepressants.[3] A compelling recent example is illustrated in an exchange of letters between the Citizens Commission for Human Rights (CCHR) and the Productivity Commission inquiry into mental health in Australia. An excerpt from the CCHR's reply to the Productivity Commission reads:

> *Your letter points to recommendations that include health screening be expanded to include 'children's social and emotional development before they enter preschool' and an 'emotional development check'. That you reject that this can be translated to mean checking for signs of 'mental illness' is semantics and misleading. Terms such as 'mental health' or 'emotional health' are now used rather than resorting to use of 'mental illness/mental health terminology'.[4]*

But it is more than just vagueness that causes confusion and compounds the deep culture of misinformation; certain terms are also used deliberately to suit specific agendas, particularly the business interests of established mental health/suicide prevention organisations profiting from the commercial opportunities of the Default Depression culture, such as delivering training programs on workplace mental health. To describe workers' experience of distress due to these workplace situations as 'mental disorder' significantly restricts how this distress, and its causes, might be addressed.[5]

Similarly, the seeming interchangeability of certain terms creates systemic confusion and diminishes the validity of research and program design and evaluation. A key example is the term 'mental health', which is used to mean a wide variety of qualitatively different things. This is further complicated by the ambiguous use of the term 'depression', especially where the terms 'depression' and 'mental health' are used interchangeably.

In general, 'mental health' refers to personal psychological and emotional wellbeing. However, as it is commonly used, the term implies the existence of its opposite – mental *ill*-health, or mental illness. This implication endorses a medicalised view of personal wellbeing – to be stress-free is to be in good mental health; conversely, to be distressed is to be symptomatic of poor mental health, or mental illness. To describe the experience of distress as 'mental illness' only adds to the community-wide confusion and ambiguity. Common terms used to describe general distress, such as 'feeling troubled', 'feeling down', 'feeling low'; or experiencing a 'loss of spirit' or loss of energy, have now become equated with 'mental health'. However these common descriptions of common human experiences should not be taken to imply a clinical mental disorder. The United Nations recognises the inherent ambiguity in terminology:

> *Terminology in the sphere of mental health is a contested terrain. There is a need to accept different terms according to how people define their own experiences of mental health. 'Mental health' itself can signal a biomedical tradition for explaining and understanding lived experiences, psychic or emotional distress, trauma, voice hearing or disability.*[6]

Acknowledging the subjective experience of distress is a crucial aspect of developing an appropriate support response. But we can't have it both ways. When we do 'accept different terms according to how people define their own experiences of mental health', we are then obliged to accept that our formal classifications might not be entirely relevant. This ambiguity is, perhaps, acceptable in everyday life; it is less acceptable in the clinical domain where there may be important impacts on a person's life.

Further ambiguity around the term 'mental health' arises from its different meanings in different contexts. It can refer to:

- general individual wellbeing and the absence of clinical disorder;
- the mental health *system* – the bureaucracy and institutions relating to *mental health*.

There is no formal oversight of workplace mental health training content. This allows the ongoing exploitation of well-meaning but misinformed workplace and human resources management who have considerable influence over workplace policy development; in their endeavours to create 'mentally healthy workplaces', people working in these capacities adopt the language and concepts of the leadership of the current approach and inadvertently perpetuate the institutionalisation of Default Depression.

The ambiguity, inconsistencies and misinformation are rampant. In a telling example, in 2019, the Prime Minister of Australia stated that 'around 80% of people who die by suicide have a mental health issue'.[7] The use of the term 'mental health issue' is as ambiguous here as elsewhere – it could mean anything from experiencing some level of distress relating to circumstances in the workplace or elsewhere in their life, to having a serious psychiatric condition. It serves little purpose other than to add to the lack of clarity and direction in this already ineffective sector. The Prime Minister's language choices reflect a broader trend. For example, the term 'mental health issues' is often cited by the media to refer to sportspeople or celebrities taking time out for personal, emotional or psychological challenges.

Throughout the literature on mental health there is a range of commonly listed mental disorders, including anxiety, mood disorders, eating disorders, and attention deficit and hyperactivity disorders. But looking at the evolving formal classification systems of mental disorders, such as DSM and ICD, it is evident that that there is a continuing trend toward medicalising more and more common human experiences; more recently, 'workplace burnout', 'prolonged' grief and 'persistent' bereavement, as well as addictions such as gaming addiction, have become classified as disorders and addictions.[8] The medicalisation of grief has been recently criticised in an article published in the *Palgrave Encyclopedia of Critical Perspectives on Mental Health*, 2022:

> *We stand at a critical juncture in the shifting landscape of how we understand grief – more specifically, how we draw the line between normal and abnormal grief and whether we should draw that line at all.*[9]

However, despite the continuing trend of developing new diagnostic classifications, far and away the most common diagnoses in mental health are depression and anxiety.

The defining characteristics and symptoms of depression and anxiety are often almost indistinguishable.[10] In other words: 'Depression and anxiety are not two disorders that coexist. They are two faces of one disorder.'[11] And they are usually treated in exactly the same way, with the prescription of the same antidepressant drugs.[12] In fact, across the second half of the 20th century, the definitions of both depression and anxiety were finessed to suit health policy and pharmaceutical development and marketing:

> *The association of anxiety with diffuse and amorphous conceptions of 'stress' and 'neuroses' became incompatible with professional norms demanding diagnostic specificity. At the same time, the contrasting nosologies [classifications] of anxiety and depression in the* Diagnostic and Statistical Manual of Mental Disorders III (DSM-III) *extended major depressive disorder to encompass far more patients than any particular anxiety disorder. In addition, antidepressant drugs were not associated with the stigma and alleged side effects of the anxiolytic [anti-anxiety]* drugs.[13]

Unhelpful ambiguity exists around the distinction between depression and anxiety as formal classification:

> *Depression and anxiety, standard psychiatric diagnoses, are part of our vocabulary and popular culture. However, these terms are employed to highlight 'idioms of distress', to describe illness*

experience and to label diagnostic categories. Their widespread, flexible and interchangeable use has blurred the boundary between distress and disease. The disease halo has been inappropriately transferred to many forms of human suffering. The medicalization of distress has resulted in a focus on treating individuals. It has also resulted in ignoring the impact of social and economic stress on mental health resulting in very little emphasis on the need for and use of public health and population-based interventions.[14]

Despite their ambiguity and the questionable research and evidence-base underpinning much of their usage, the terms 'depression', 'anxiety' and 'mental health' nevertheless dominate planning and activity designed to address people in psychological and emotional distress.

An important example of this is the association of mental illness with suicide; unquestioned preoccupation with this tenuous association undermines effective suicide prevention efforts, because, according to an article published in *Frontiers in Public Health* (2022), 'the majority of people who die by suicide have never seen a mental health professional or been diagnosed with a mental illness'.[15]

This unfounded belief, built on widespread myths, misinformation and core conceptualisation and ideas (such as the biomedical model and the process of medicalisation), fully pervades the mental health sector, and has become the dominant conceptual framework on which government and organisational policy and practice is built.

Pathologising and medicalising human distress

People suffer psychological distress at different times in their lives and for different reasons. This sort of common suffering may be described as 'a state of emotional suffering associated with stressors and demands that are difficult to cope with in daily life'.[16] This suffering is not pathological or abnormal; it is the understandable human response to stressful circumstances. Most healthy people experience this sort of distress at some point in their life.

As UN Special Rapporteur Dainius Pūras, in his *Report of the Right of Everyone to the Enjoyment of the Highest Attainable Standard of Physical and Mental Health*, stated in 2020:

> *Current mental health policies have been affected to a large extent by the asymmetry of power and biases because of the dominance of the biomedical model and biomedical interventions. This model has led ... to the medicalization of normal reactions to life's many pressures, including moderate forms of social anxiety, sadness, shyness, truancy and antisocial behaviour. The most vocal message that can reach stakeholders with the resources and power to support meaningful transformation in global mental health is the need to close the 'treatment gap'. The Special Rapporteur is concerned that this message may further the excessive use of diagnostic categories and expand the medical model to diagnose pathologies and provide individual treatment modalities that lead to excessive medicalization. The message diverts policies and practices from embracing two powerful modern approaches: a public health approach and a human rights-based approach.*[17]

This complements work by Dr John Ashfield, a UK practitioner in palliative care, and his colleagues.

> *Perhaps there is a problem with the way we have come to define and respond to personal distress – including psychological and emotional difficulties, which previously would not have been the domain of medical intervention and diagnosis, and would have been largely resolved with various forms of non-medical human support. Augmenting this idea with some closer analysis of the mental health 'industry', what we discover, contrary to what we have been told so often, is not a crisis of mental ill-health at all, but the effects of a deeply flawed narrative of 'mental illness', directly related to the systematic medicalisation of common human experience. Put simply, a whole gamut of common, albeit sometimes very challenging and disconcerting human experience, has been corralled by medicine (and in particular its specialty of psychiatry) and referred to as*

illness; and where there is illness, treatments and especially drugs are utilised to attempt to cure it.[18]

In Australia, medicalisation exists though all sectors, including the Australian Government, who offer confused advice on mental health with the conflation of *mental or behavioural condition* with *mental illness* and imply that depression and anxiety are an illness.

Mental health in Australia: a quick guide

When a person has a condition that affects their mental health, they may have a mental illness or mental health disorder. This includes conditions such as depression, anxiety, schizophrenia and bipolar disorder.

The most recent ABS National Health Survey estimated there were 4.8 million Australians (20.1 per cent) with a mental or behavioural condition in 2017–18.[19]

Why mental illness labelling is problematic

The problematic nature of mental illness labelling has been vigorously debated in literature.[20] One of the great and perhaps tragic ironies of the conceptualisation and messaging of the whole mental health/suicide prevention sector is that while there is a focus on de-stigmatisation of mental illness, as much as anything, it is actually the language and labelling at the core of the current approach that creates and perpetuates the stigma. Ashfield and his colleagues have discussed this at length, and it is worth reproducing some of it here:

It is important to take a moment to consider not only the medical conceptualisation of human experience as illness, and the burgeoning use of psychoactive drug treatments, but as well the influence of illness language itself. Words are not merely descriptive, as one might imagine, they are causative, and can have unexpected consequences. There is a saying, 'give a person a label and soon they'll begin to live up to it'. Unnecessarily naming and defining common human experience (however difficult) as 'illness' or 'disorder' can modify the way people perceive themselves (and how others see them and respond to them) and may affect their self-confidence, self-image, and subsequent life choices, negatively. Put plainly, this kind of language serves no positive purpose, and may harm people; yet it is central to mental health literacy content.

Consider the following common trajectory and its compounding factors: an individual reports their experience of distress to a doctor who feels obliged to provide a diagnosis of some kind of disorder (most commonly an affective disorder), a script for medication, and perhaps a referral to a mental health practitioner, requiring a Mental Health Treatment Plan. Factors that may compound this potentially negative trajectory, may, as already mentioned, include: a change in self-perception, and in the way that others (such as work colleagues, friends, and family) perceive their diagnosis. The individual may take time off work for recovery, and withdraw from some social responsibilities and socially inclusive activities, further reinforcing their illness status and trajectory. It must be considered here that such compounding factors have potential to create a subtle yet consequential shift from an internal locus of control to an external one: unwitting acquiescence to an illness entity and to those (professionals) who have the only means by which to treat it.[21]

Chapter 9

Proposing new language

Developing a more effective approach to issues of mental health and suicide will depend upon the introduction of appropriate language and terminology, without resorting to pathologising language.

The term 'psychological distress' is an example, as Tina Arvidsdotter et al. stated in an article published in the *Scandinavian Journal of Caring Sciences* in 2015:

> Struggling to cope with everyday life, Feeling inferior to others *and* Losing one's grip on life. *It seems to be associated with a gradual depletion of existential capacities and lead[s] to dissatisfaction, suffering, poor self-esteem and lack of control. As psychological distress may be a forerunner to mental, physical and emotional exhaustion, there is a need to initiate preventive or early interventions to avoid mental, physical and emotional chaos in such patients. Patients' with psychological distress need to be involved in a person-centred salutogenic [health-giving] dialogue with health professionals to become aware of and strengthen their own capacities to regain health and wellbeing.*[1]

The term 'psychological distress' is an acceptable alternative to help understand and describe the dimensions of distress without medicalisation, and consequently provides a starting point to more effectively consider and deal with distress.[2] The following definitions fit with that approach, as Dr John Ashfield explains:

The severity of this [mental health] difficulty can be registered as either a low intensity mental health difficulty *or a* high intensity mental health difficulty, *thus avoiding the words disorder and illness altogether. This substitution of language may preserve people's dignity by avoiding harmful labelling, at the same time avoiding trivialising complex difficulties – the experience of which may on occasions be acutely painful, profoundly distressing, debilitating, or disruptive.*[3]

Our collective understanding of key terms and definitions needs to be clear and consistent if our prevention efforts are to be effective. This book responds to this need and presents a new set of terms and definitions consistent with the best available current thinking and data. This chapter includes a number of these new terms and definitions; a full set has been included as an appendix to help facilitate the use of new and more appropriate language (*see* Appendix D: Appropriate language for suicide prevention and the mental health sector).

The Situational Approach

The Situational Approach to suicide prevention challenges fundamental aspects of the current suicide prevention paradigm, including its individualistic nature that (a) individuals in distress have a mental disorder that can be diagnosed and treated medically, and (b) their social context is largely irrelevant to this process. The Situational Approach regards the broader social context, including personal relationships, family background and employment, as fundamentally important to the psychological or emotional wellbeing of the individual. Two complementary concepts are the 'biopsychosocial' approach, and the social determinants of health/ mental health.[4]

For the most part these concepts are similar and complement each other. One important distinction is the Situational Approach acknowledges that there are times when some individuals suffer 'high intensity mental health difficulties', such as schizophrenic or psychotic experiences, with no social causal correlate.[5] But even in this context, Ashfield and his colleagues warn:

Every suicide death has a situational context.

Regarding suicide prevention: People living in distress with high intensity mental health difficulties, even where there appears to be no external or social causal correlate that can be identified, need their situational context to be considered as a priority for their ongoing care and support. Situational contexts such as: their family and relationship contexts, finances, health service availability and employment/employability are all crucially important to their ongoing wellbeing.

The University of Rochester Medical Center in the United States describes the biopsychosocial approach as an approach that 'systematically considers biological, psychological, and social factors and their complex interactions in understanding health, illness, and health care delivery'.[6]

The Situational Approach[7] to suicide prevention acknowledges the predominant link between *situational distress* and suicide. It is principally informed by, and responds to, risk factors of a broad spectrum of difficult human experiences throughout one's life. The simple fact is that for all suicide deaths, the situational context has had a significant influence in the tragic path that has been taken. Appropriate and effective support for their wellbeing cannot be considered without that social context being central to their ongoing care. This approach is also mindful of – and wherever possible seeks to address – contextual, systemic, and socio-cultural risk and protective factors and determinants: the real world of individuals' lived experience.[8] The Situational Approach looks at how to provide appropriate support for these distressed people, and to minimise the cause of the distress.

The Situational Approach offers a sound conceptual framework for more effective prevention, and challenges key tenets of the ineffectual current biomedical approach, which views psychological distress as symptomatic of a disorder or illness of some kind requiring diagnosis and treatment. This individualised approach reinforces the assumption of a disordered organism/brain, and pathologising and medicalising common human experience. It corrals the bulk of psychological distress into the diagnostic category of *affective disorders* with numerous sub-categories of depression and anxiety; all commonly referred to as 'disorders' or 'illnesses'. In this paradigm, depression in particular is associated with suicide not as a possible correlate but, by implication, as a causal factor. The conflation of so-called 'mental illness' with suicide continues to be a prime reason for the failure of so many enterprises of suicide prevention, because it diverts attention away from the more situational and contextual course of most suicides.

The following tables of terms and definitions are presented as an introductory model. They offer suggestions for new and more appropriate terminology for use in addressing the challenges of mental health and suicide. The tables have been built on work already done from a variety of sources, with modifications where necessary. The terms and definitions are not meant to be considered exhaustive or final; they are expected to evolve as the Situational Approach becomes more firmly entrenched as a suitable conceptual framework for the mental health/suicide prevention sector. As mentioned, a more comprehensive set of terms and definitions can be found as a standalone resource document at Appendix D.

Table 1. Key terms

Situational distress	Situational distress encompasses a significantly challenging or troubling experience of thoughts, emotions, bodily sensations, or behaviours, associated with difficult life events, such as bereavement, a change in health status, relationship breakdown, financial, or occupational difficulties. This distress may significantly overlap with many of the symptoms usually taken to suggest mental disorders (such as depression and anxiety).[9]
	The conceptual basis for situational distress acknowledges social determinants such as unemployment, and financial and relationship difficulties, as having a key role as causal factors in distress. However, sometimes in cases of acute distress, there are no evident social causal factors, such as with some high-intensity mental health difficulties like schizophrenic or other psychotic experiences. Notwithstanding, the situational context remains a vitally important consideration. In the case of suicidality and death by suicide, the situational context is also a vital consideration. Regardless of the causal factors involved, people in extreme distress need their situational context – including family context, finances, health/mental health and community support services availability – to be considered as a priority for appropriate responses and ongoing care and support.
Psychological distress	Psychological distress refers to patterns of psychological and emotional discomfort and general unpleasant feelings and emotions. It is an umbrella term to describe some common interrelated identifiable patterns of difficulty including stress, insomnia, depression, anxiety and suicidal thoughts. Psychological distress may be associated with factors such as: interpersonal difficulties, bereavement, lack of sleep, use of drugs or alcohol, workplace stress or abuse and physical illness.
	Some of the most potent factors associated with psychological distress are thoughts and feelings of powerlessness. For distressed individuals, feeling powerless, and perceiving themselves to be powerless, can result in a decline in general mental capacity (thinking, problem solving, and memory recall), irritability, anger, and diminished verbal communication.[10] The stress of this experience can trigger multi-system changes in the body,[11] further compounding the difficulties an individual may face. Although people suffering psychological distress may experience a great deal of difficulty in their general mental capacity, this should not be presumed to be a psychiatric disorder or illness.

| High intensity psychological distress | **High-intensity psychological distress** refers to acute psychological and emotional distress which may require direct supportive intervention. People suffering high intensity psychological distress may be at elevated risk of suicide.[12]

This level of distress usually significantly impairs a person's ability to function on a day-to-day basis and noticeably interferes with their usual or preferred mental, emotional, or social capacity, and their experience of feeling capable and competent.

Distress of this intensity often requires more than a person's own coping ability, lifestyle adjustments, and support of friends and family. At least initially, it may require thoughtful observation and reflective assessment by a qualified health professional (a doctor, psychotherapist, psychologist, or, in some cases, a psychiatrist), who may also suggest appropriate psychotherapy (psychological therapy).

It is important to understand that having experiences such as schizophrenia or psychotic episodes does not necessarily make a person suicidal, and that, with the right support, people who have these experiences can live a satisfactory and manageable life.[13] In this regard, the World Health Organization (WHO) emphasises psychosocial interventions as particularly important support strategies.[14]

The term 'high intensity psychological distress' is proposed as a less pathologising alternative to the commonly used but restrictive and ambiguous terms such as **mental disorder** or **mental illness**. |
| Self-harm | **Self-harm refers** to deliberate self-injury or other physical harm such as cutting, burning, poisoning, or overdosing on drugs (including prescription medications) and/or alcohol.

Self-harm is common, and not only among teenagers.[15] However, it is crucial to note that, in most cases, self-harm is not an attempt at suicide and does not lead to suicide.[16]

The relationship between suicide and self-harm is complicated. People with a history of self-harm are at considerably higher risk of suicide.[17] However, there is some evidence, including a Finnish study[18] and an American study,[19] that many, perhaps the majority, of suicide deaths occur on the first attempt.

Although there is some overlap between people who attempt but do not complete suicide and those who do complete suicide, these groups are characterised by significant demographic and clinical differences.[20]

Most cases of self-harm occur in females, as do most cases of attempted but incomplete suicide; but most suicide deaths occur in males.[21] In many cases of self-harm, there is a history of behavioural difficulties, substance misuse, and family, social, and psychological problems.[22] None of this should be automatically presumed to indicate a mental disorder.

Self-harm should always be taken seriously, whether or not the intention is suicide. |

There is a situational context relevant to every suicide death. Very often, there is substantial situational distress in the preceding days, weeks, months, or even years.

Extensive research shows that many people who kill themselves have no history of mental disorder and/or are impacted by difficult social circumstances.[23] The majority of people who kill themselves have been in circumstances likely to cause enormous stress in their lives, such as unemployment – the majority of all suicide deaths in Australia are people of working age who were not employed at the time of their death.[24] It is crucial that this issue be considered as a priority in current and future suicide prevention planning and initiatives.

People suffering high intensity psychological distress (see definition above) may be at elevated risk of suicide. This distress is often associated with difficult social and financial circumstances which may precipitate a state of despair or hopelessness. Such people may be greatly in need of and may benefit from timely and competent professional support. Regardless of the associated factors, it may further compound the difficulties being faced by people in distress to reduce the scope of support solely to health/mental health professionals.

Many people who die by suicide have recently engaged with a mental health professional.[25] Limiting preventive strategies to those built upon the presumption of mental disorder or illness will simply not help many, perhaps the majority, of people at risk of suicide. There is also evidence showing that inappropriate support can discourage people away from seeking help again.[26] Effective suicide prevention requires that measures of prevention are non-pathologising, informed by evidence-based, gender-specific differences in help seeking, and part of a broader, more encompassing approach that takes account of social determinants.

Risk factors and protective factors

Suicide prevention activity should be informed by known risk factors and protective factors. There are many known risk factors associated with stress in a person's life that may contribute/lead to suicide. It is important for effective suicide prevention that we design and target prevention activities according to the prevalence and strength of the risk factors in different demographic groups.

Risk and protective factors for psychological or emotional wellbeing act at several different levels, consequently responses to these factors need to be multi-layered and multi-sectoral. Health, education, welfare, transport, and housing sectors are all crucially important and need to be involved at the core of any preventive activity. It is important that these key agencies outside health/mental health have a vital leadership role in suicide prevention rather than just as a superficial 'partner' to health/mental health in order to fulfil token inter-agency requirements.

Table 2. Risk factors and protective factors

At-risk	In general, **at-risk** refers to individuals and groups who have higher rates of suicide compared with the general population. Identifying people at-risk can play an important role in helping focus preventive activities.
Risk factors	**Risk factors** are factors that may negatively impact on a person's life and experience in a way that potentially increases the likelihood of suicide. Key risk factors for suicide include social determinants such as unemployment, financial difficulties and homelessness, as well as high intensity psychological difficulties (such as some psychiatric conditions), prior suicide attempts, alcohol misuse, serious health challenges, childhood abuse, psychological trauma, grief, separation and divorce, and the experience of powerlessness. Risk factors vary relative to age, gender, and other intersecting social and cultural factors. However, the evidence suggests that in many, and perhaps the majority of cases, multiple risk factors combine to elevate psychological distress to intolerable levels. Several risk factors may be influential at multiple levels and may overlap.[27]

The spectrum of suicide prevention activity

Currently, suicide prevention initiatives reflect two broadly different orientations and approaches, which need to be reconciled in relation to both their effectiveness, and potential complementarity.[28] The different models can generally be broken down into:

- a broadscale, population-wide perspective targeting individuals who may be acutely distressed and at-risk, also known as 'upstream' prevention,
- and direct intervention with those identified as at-risk, or already in crisis, and the follow-up support for people affected by suicide, also known as 'downstream' prevention.

Much of the current approach to suicide prevention sits within the downstream, acute level of intervention. While important in dealing with those identified as being of elevated risk, the acute level of intervention misses many people who kill themselves, and thus cannot be expected to reduce the overall toll of suicide deaths. This is then compounded by ineffectual upstream activity, where the largest funding is directed to organisations and activity that perpetuate the current approach.

Table 3. Prevention levels and strategies

Upstream prevention	**Upstream prevention** addresses financial, environmental, industrial and economic structures and conditions that may impact negatively on the wellbeing of individuals in the overall population or population subgroups.
	Effective upstream prevention activity is required to reduce the overall toll of suicide deaths. To be effective, upstream prevention activity should address fundamental social and economic structures that can enable improved social support and general protective factors across the total population. This can be done through appropriate broadscale public health and health promotion activity, in which health professionals can take an advocacy role in interagency work with key government departments and activity such as housing and infrastructure.
	This level or type of activity is distinct from the later, intervention and postvention (or downstream prevention), activity which tends to focus on individuals. Common current upstream prevention activities include public awareness campaigns, community outreach services, and community education.
	Key factors in suicide deaths such as unemployment, financial difficulties, and housing insecurity often cause intense distress. Appropriate population-level interventions to support people experiencing these challenges should primarily focus on activity outside the health/mental health sector, such as job-creation, re-employment support, housing affordability policies, and financial support programs.

Downstream prevention	**Downstream prevention** refers to activity that is generally limited to dealing directly with individuals who have been identified as at-risk of suicide, and/or ongoing postvention support (e.g. counselling/psychotherapy) for family and friends affected by suicide and suicidality.
	Although downstream prevention is vitally important in caring for highly distressed individuals, it cannot play a major role in reducing the overall toll of suicide deaths. This is in large part because many people who die by suicide do not have meaningful engagement, if any engagement at all, with health/support services prior to their death
Public health interventions	**Public health interventions** are population-wide approaches by the health sector, often in collaboration with other sectors, including housing, employment, education, and transport.
	Appropriate public health activity built on good research and planning represents an important opportunity to effectively address the suicide death toll. However, public health activity in the mental health/suicide prevention sector (and the health sector more broadly) has tended to reflect a narrow focus on a medicalised approach, and where there have been attempts to advocate to broaden the focus to include social determinants such as poverty and housing, there has generally not been the political will to enact this in any substantial way.[29]
Acute intervention	**Acute intervention** refers to engagement by health/welfare workers with individuals who are already so highly psychologically distressed they are at a greater risk of self-harm or suicide.
	Ideally, acute intervention would occur in broader settings than just the medical/mental health domain, and should include all relevant government agencies (such as housing and employment support) as well as not-for-profit and community care organisations.
	It is important at the individual level, but it has limited preventive impact at the population level.[30]
Crisis intervention	Like acute intervention, **crisis intervention** refers to engaging directly with individuals who are at high risk of imminent self-harm or suicide.
Suicide postvention	**Suicide postvention** refers to follow-up support for people affected by a suicide death or incomplete attempted suicide. Suicide postvention may include grief counselling and preventive support for family and friends of individuals who have died by suicide.
	This support is vitally important, because family and friends may be at increased risk of suicide themselves, because of their responses to the suicide (e.g. grief and/or guilt). However, like any other later intervention, postvention is limited in its scope of prevention, because it generally only targets people who have been identified by health/support services as being at-risk through their connection to individual suicide deaths or incomplete suicide attempts.

Table 4. Clarification of some key terms and concepts

Rates versus numbers	Both rates and numbers of suicide deaths are important for consideration of appropriate suicide prevention activity. However, either considered alone without reference to the other can give a distorted representation of suicide deaths. Rates of suicide are generally measured as deaths per 100,000 of a population group.[31] However, although this facilitates comparisons between different groups, it can give rise to a skewed representation when working with relatively small populations such as in rural areas in Australia. High rates in a small population may justify specific targeted interventions, but this may not lead to a reduction in the overall toll if larger populations with larger numbers of suicide deaths but lower rates are not properly targeted as well. Numbers are simply the total numbers of deaths in an area or group. For larger population areas, relatively large numbers of suicide deaths may be reported/expressed as a relatively lower rate and consequently not receive the attention they deserve.
Gender specificity in suicide prevention	The suicide death/self-harm spectrum is strongly gender-specific. Although there is some overlap, the large majority (about 75%) of suicide deaths occur in males, but the large majority of incidents of non-fatal self-harm occur in females.[32] To develop effective preventive activity on this suicide/self-harm spectrum requires clearly defined, evidence-based gender-specific activity on a scale proportionate to the risk level of the target group
Rural versus metropolitan	In general, rural rates of suicide are higher than in metropolitan areas. However, the great majority of Australian suicide deaths occur in city-dwelling adults.[33] This is not a contradiction: there are high rates of suicide in many rural areas of Australia, and the development of appropriate preventive activity is required to address this. And although rural rates of suicide are generally higher than metropolitan rates, this is a considerable generalisation: rates vary enormously if measured by locality (for example, local government areas or federal electorates) in both rural and metropolitan areas.[34] Some metropolitan areas have both higher rates of suicide than many rural areas and considerably higher numbers of suicide deaths than many rural areas. The five capital cities of Sydney, Melbourne, Brisbane, Adelaide and Perth together account for over half (54.18%) of all suicide deaths in Australia. Suicide rates tend to be higher in socially and economically disadvantaged areas.[35] Note: Torrens University Australia hosts a very good online suicide mapping tool: **Torrens University Australia Public Health Information Development Unit** (PHIDU) Social Health Atlases. The website hosts interactive maps on health data, including suicide, in multiple geographical areas.

| Self-harm versus first-time attempt | Although there is some overlap between people who attempt suicide and those who complete suicide, these groups are characterised by significant demographic and clinical differences.[36] Although people who intentionally self-harm (including incomplete suicide attempts) have an elevated risk of going on to kill themselves, the majority do not do so.[37] The best available evidence suggests that the majority of completed suicides are first-time attempts.[38] |

Depression and anxiety

Despite many suicides deaths having no evidence of prior mental disorder, and the strong place of adverse life events in suicide deaths, much of the current approach continues to push the paradigm of illness and mental deficiency and the unhelpful focus on categories of mental disorder.

| Depression | There is an enormous body of published literature questioning not just the role of depression in suicide deaths but also key aspects of the conceptualisation of depression. The experience of being human can sometimes be acutely distressing, even overwhelming and debilitating. Nevertheless, such experience does not necessarily constitute a diagnosable mental illness, and in fact is often a normal response to stressful events such as financial difficulties, workplace problems, or housing problems. |
| Anxiety disorder | Anxiety is a perfectly natural human experience. It is a reaction to stress that has both psychological and physical features. Some experts consider that stress, anxiety, and depression are different aspects of the same psychological distress, and that making a distinction between anxiety and depression is unhelpful. Anxiety levels for some people may become overwhelming and chronic, with a debilitating impact on their daily lives, and they may need treatment. However, anxiety should not be automatically presumed to be a mental disorder. Causes of the stress should always be considered in supporting people with anxiety. |

Chapter 10

What we need for more effective suicide prevention in Australia

It is a national shame and an abuse of the good intentions of so many working and volunteering in our suicide prevention sector to continue funding organisations that have been ineffective over a long period of time. Why continue to throw large amounts of money into a system that offers no return? It serves only to reinforce the status and profile of organisations whose business agendas directly conflict with the needs of the community. Despite the best of intentions, many workers and volunteers in this sector unwittingly endorse and perpetuate the established narrative around mental health and the Default Depression response to distress.

We face enormous obstacles. This book is directly challenging well-funded, well-entrenched organisations; a systemic, bureaucratised approach to suicide and distress that is largely built on the narrative of distress as mental illness, with a major but unhelpful over-emphasis on depression, and deeply held and widespread beliefs that support this approach. Nevertheless, we must begin somewhere. We can take some guidance from the UN:

we should not accept that medications and other biomedical interventions be commonly used to address issues which are closely related to social problems, unequal power relationships, violence and other adversities that determine our social and emotional environment. There is a need of a shift in investments in mental health, from focusing on 'chemical imbalances' to focusing on 'power imbalances' and inequalities.[1]

So, how might we begin this shift and become more effective?

For a start, we need re-invigorated and broadened leadership. Clearly, the current leadership has not produced the outcomes that might reasonably be expected from their huge budgets – in fact, the current leadership has become a significant part of the problem.

Caution is required: addressing the challenges that come with the current leadership is not just a matter of consulting or partnering with that leadership and expecting or hoping they might accommodate new ideas. They have been avoiding or discounting criticism for at least a decade and a half; for example, by offering token acknowledgement of issues such as the role of social determinants, or writing a new position statement about factors such as unemployment, or men and suicide but, in reality, not following up with anything substantial or evidence based. They offer token responses to mollify genuine concerns while further reinforcing their own business structures and processes.

We need the integrity to openly acknowledge the unhelpful and even harmful nature of much of the current approach to suicide prevention and mental health, which has consistently disregarded the expertise of senior academics, researchers and other experts who offer contrasting opinions. As it stands, the current discourse offers limited scope for the serious and open discussion needed to begin to address the inherent deficits of the current approach. We now have a well-established network of organisations in the mental health/ suicide prevention sector throughout Australia. This network could facilitate the transition to more effective work in this sector – with the important proviso: we need to implement a major national professional development program to ensure competency in understanding a new and more appropriate approach to suicide prevention and personal wellbeing. Many well-meaning personnel throughout the country who work and volunteer in suicide prevention have a sense of the limits of the current system and understand the need to broaden our ideas about prevention and support – however, the current system is so deeply entrenched that despite the good intentions to try to provide appropriate support from outside the medical system, many people in distress still end up being directed into the limiting pathway of the health/mental health system.

The human resources sector is a prime example: regardless of the literature and efforts of community suicide prevention to look more broadly for answers, human resources policies and procedures are structured so that they have little option but to direct distressed workers toward a GP, and the almost inevitable medicalised processing.

Individual organisations within this network need to be prepared to:

- put aside their endorsement (either implicit or explicit) of the leadership of the current approach;
- end their partnerships with organisations perpetuating the paradigm of illness and deficiency in mental health;
- develop new priorities according to a more appropriate approach to suicide prevention and to begin practising accordingly.

Underpinning this, we need a new set of messages for the community, including the central message that the experience of distress does not automatically mean the existence of a clinical mental disorder.

The impact of Default Depression on our overall political, social, and business and industrial culture extends far beyond just the health/ mental health, general human services and welfare sectors. However, one of the sectors most compromised by the nature of the current approach is suicide prevention.

The ideas presented in this chapter are presented as starting points only. Hopefully, motivated activists will develop each section further as templates for action.

A fully funded multi-year program of activity

A major symposium considering the Situational Approach was held in Sydney in 2018 and featured participants from all over Australia.[2] The gathering demonstrated that there is already a collective of senior industry representatives and academics, people with lived experience, politicians and community-level activists who may be willing and able to establish a high-level steering committee to oversee a comprehensive transition to a more effective and appropriate system of suicide prevention and support for people in acute distress or crisis. Senior personnel from the insurance industry, along with senior academics, have been advocating for the establishment of a new organisation to facilitate change toward the Situational Approach within the finance sector – this could easily be expanded in scope to oversee wholesale change across the mental health/suicide prevention sector.

It is crucial that this transition is integrated at all levels and throughout all relevant sectors. Once the fundamental conceptual framework, the culture of this work, and the knowledge and training changes, much of the community-level activity, and the skills of the personnel currently involved, could be transitioned to more effective work in this sector.

There are more than enough willing people to begin a nationwide program of activity that more fully accommodates the breadth of the available evidence and offers a good chance of slowing the escalating toll of suicide deaths, diagnoses of mental disorders, and prescribing of antidepressants.

We must lobby governments, industry and community leaders to collaboratively adopt a Situational Approach to suicide prevention and personal wellbeing.

New leadership and expertise

For some time, there have been openly expressed concerns about key individuals and organisations of the current leadership.[3] The recent recommendation by the Productivity Commission to screen children aged from birth to three years old for their mental health clearly shows how out-of-touch this leadership is.[4] There are serious ethical concerns about this astonishing and entirely inappropriate recommendation for a number of reasons, including the lack of evidence base for the proposed screening and the potentially harmful outcomes, for example, from harsh antidepressant medication.

We need expertise and new, informed leadership to steer policy development, funding allocation, research, organisational change and community program activity toward a completely revitalised, more effective system of suicide prevention. This new leadership should be engaged across all relevant settings and sectors including the health/mental health system, welfare and support services, research and industry, and the workplace generally. Suicide prevention activities and clinical services of the mental health system and its professionals overlap; in some cases, individuals experiencing high-intensity psychological distress associated with suicidal ideation or self-harm may require clinical intervention. Thus the health/mental health system will continue to have a role. Nonetheless, many distressed individuals do not have a diagnosable clinical mental or psychiatric condition, so suicide prevention activities need to occur outside of the clinical remit of health/mental health services. A broader field of suicide prevention expertise will include:

- knowledge of population health and social determinants; mental health-related epidemiology
- social research and research analysis
- knowledge specific to relevant agencies and services (including housing, legal and employment); how to effectively work as key agents in suicide prevention
- knowledge of workplace activities in mental health and suicide prevention, and how collaborative partnerships can be formed
- workplace training – networks, accreditation
- knowledge of the role of GPs and psychiatrists in the current provision of mental health services
- community development and health promotion, built on creditable local evidence
- knowledge of male psychology (which reaches beyond popular but often simplistic and unhelpful notions of male behaviour) and male-specific group work
- adult education

- knowledge of the health/mental health system, and Common-wealth primary health network companies and their preferred providers of psychological and mental health services.

To ensure new activity is not compromised to suit the business agendas of current high-profile organisations, we need separation from the existing leadership, as explained by Ashfield and Smith:

> *Current suicide prevention and 'mental health' literacy thinking, and initiatives (exhibited by government and non-government organisations), have tended to be informed by a quite narrow field of expertise exclusively derivative of the status quo mental illness ideology, affecting policy, research, program design, and service delivery approaches. Hence the imperative of comprehensive change involving a much broader field of experts, disciplines, and perspectives, and one that places a premium on innovation that is preventative rather than oriented to late intervention and crisis intervention, most characteristic of current approaches.*
>
> *The breadth of expertise and leadership needed to take us beyond the current mental illness status quo that so impoverishes efforts of effective suicide prevention and that of psychological well-being and mental health promotion, will encompass:*
> - *research knowledge and experience that is referenced to a broad evidence base and broader perspective than the present illness ideology*
> - *community engagement and development*
> - *communications, mass media expertise*
> - *partnership brokerage*
> - *marketing*
> - *gender differences pertinent to intentionally non-fatal self-harm, suicide, and mental health difficulties.*[5]

New leadership can facilitate the development of a new vision and set of priorities for action, as well as consulting with government and other organisations to help develop a fresh set of policies to ensure activity in the mental health/suicide prevention sector is accountable to the newly developed priorities and policies.

The last decade and a half at least have shown that without substantial change to the leadership, good intention will be swallowed up in newly written plans that do no more than perpetuate the assumed authority of that leadership.

Competent personnel in human services beyond the health/mental health sector

Ashfield and Smith advocate for a fresh approach in their paper *The Situational Approach to Suicide Prevention and Mental Health Literacy: Advocating for a new multi-sector and multidisciplinary approach*:

> It is vital that suicide prevention and mental health literacy initiatives are informed afresh by expertise beyond our present mental health system and its underpinning assumptions. Already our proposed Situational Approach is gaining currency as a useful conceptualisation of a new approach to both these endeavours. However, for systemic and effective change to occur, a broad church of professional collaboration will be needed – including people with knowledge and skill-sets that have not always been co-opted for these endeavours – such as professionals with expertise in finance, vocational guidance, accommodation, relationship counselling and human services support.[6]

People with lived experience

There are plenty of people across Australia with lived experience who have the skills and passion to take leadership roles at all levels, as well as acting in advisory capacity at senior government and corporate levels – and who are fully supportive of the need to adopt the Situational Approach. Direct experience and insight into the challenges of situational distress should be at the centre of discourse and planning of the transition to more effective, community-based action.

Community activists

Respected, highly competent community activists, with a history of integrity in voicing concern about the current approach, have been effectively sidelined from funding opportunities to implement more appropriate support at the community level. Funding requirements determine that community prevention activities are generally designed so that they suit the business agendas of leadership organisations of the sector. These power dynamics need to be reconsidered. It is important to break down the current arbitrary distinction between 'bureaucracies' and 'the community' in determining what types of 'mental health/suicide prevention' activities draw available funding. The settings for new community-level leadership must extend to and include the management level for health, other government agencies and not-for-profits.

People working in the mental health/suicide prevention sector

Like the community activists described above, there are plenty of people with prevention expertise in the mental health/suicide prevention sector who are open for the need to change. They are well placed to lead change toward more effective ways of dealing with distress and suicide prevention. As noted earlier – expertise is needed in more *upstream* prevention, rather than the more *downstream intervention* and *postvention* activities.

Senior academics/researchers

Respected senior academics and researchers, both nationally and internationally, can help facilitate the comprehensive change needed in the mental health/suicide prevention sector, and the relevant human services. While the current leadership has enjoyed their profile and privilege over the last decade or two, others have been working diligently to challenge key aspects of the current approach and have the requisite skills and knowledge to contribute to a more effective approach.

Nationwide professional development

To ensure appropriate workforce education and quality program design and implementation, we need a national, comprehensive professional development program. This will require large budgets – but these budgets are already in place and only need to be redirected from the current funding recipients to more suitable providers, with a possibility of return for that investment. The current approach is throwing large amounts of money into a system that offers no return. Professional development is needed in:

- the health/mental health sector, including GP training, to ensure that GPs understand a Situational Approach to suicide prevention, and to more effectively identify people at risk due to situational or social factors rather than 'mental disorders'
- the broader relevant human services, including welfare agencies and crisis support services, to ensure management and staff throughout the welfare and support services sector are appropriately skilled; that they understand that prevention activity should be largely directed at the causes of distress rather than directing people into the health/mental health system and that, if or when it is needed, staff can respond with appropriate support and/or referral
- human resources to ensure their personnel understand they have an important role in redressing the entrenchment of Default Depression in organisational policy and practice
- media to hold journalists and media organisations accountable for their perpetuation of the current narrative around mental illness.

To move toward normalising and contextualising human distress through media, policy development, research and program planning and design, we must ensure social determinants of distress are at the forefront of prevention activity.

Targeted, evidence-based community activity

Rather than maintaining and supporting the unhelpful aspects of the current approach, such as continuing to focus on depression and treatment for mental disorders to the exclusion of addressing the major evidence-based social determinants of distress, we need to direct community activity toward effective prevention.

Community engagement that brings community members together to discuss and become involved in local suicide prevention initiatives will ensure the broader Situational Approach – rather than the narrative built around mental illness – is the accepted framework for planning community activity.

Within this, there is an opportunity to promote and replicate functioning models already in place, some of which, outlined here, fit clearly with the principles of the Situational Approach.

The Safe Haven Cafe

The Safe Haven Cafe in Aldershot, UK, is a pilot project that aims to provide appropriate, wraparound support for people in crisis.[7] The cafe partners with a range of sectors to improve the system of care for people in crisis and to help find them the support they need, whatever their circumstances. Overseen by an operational steering committee, the cafe's key aim is to reduce the medical emphasis in acute care (where possible, the project avoids the use of the term 'mental illness'), and to recognise the benefits of peer support and other third-sector (that is, community) providers in helping manage a crisis.

Mt Druitt Shed

The Mt Druitt Shed in Western Sydney provides support to people who may be at risk of serious stress and suicide, generally on account of cumulative stress due to disadvantaged situations.[8] Most of the clients are men and are of Aboriginal and Torres Strait Islander origin, although the service support provided is not exclusive to men; women often find the support they need there as well. The project has been funded since 2004 by the Commonwealth Department of Health and

Ageing through the National Strategy for Prevention of Suicide. The workers at the Shed consider the circumstances of the individual clients and direct them to the assigned personnel from the relevant human services, including housing, employment and legal and financial services. Complementing this process, a range of service providers engage with people at the Shed to facilitate supportive engagement, including Probation and Parole and mental health services.

> *The Shed is easily physically described but what it is, is more complicated. Officially it is a men's suicide prevention/drop-in centre with a focus on Aboriginal and Torres Strait Islander men who have been in prison. But a lot of men don't go there for counselling in the traditional sense, and they don't go there because they are having suicidal thoughts.*
>
> *Some go there because they are homeless and want a meal. Or they need Legal Aid support. Or help with Centrelink forms. At the Shed men can find lawyers, Centrelink officers, parole officers, even a podiatrist. Some go there because they want a chat and they trust the men at The Shed. It also welcomes women.[9]*

The success of the Shed was formally acknowledged when it won the Aboriginal Justice Award in 2017.[10] A Report from Western Sydney University describes the importance of the personal connections that are developed at the Shed and the impact this has.

> *Of course, we cannot 'prove' that the drop in suicide rates in the area should be attributed directly to the Shed. But we can say with conviction that we have learned how to connect many men who need mental health services with appropriate provision, men who would otherwise not have had this access. Likewise, on a daily basis, the Shed workers 'walk with' men and their families through serious challenges, which we know, if not addressed, can lead on downward spiralling paths of despair and even suicide.[11]*

The Centre for Male Health – Western Sydney University shows a video on their Facebook page that illustrates the variety of services and support that the Shed provides from the perspectives of participants and service providers.[12] The success of the interagency connection has enabled the Shed to support a growing number of women.

Community Alliance Program

The authors of the Situational Approach have developed a number of training programs suitable for professional development at all levels, as well as for community information sessions. These programs, built on the evidence base of the Situational Approach, have been developed from highly successful community programs and could be modified to suit different sectors and contexts.

GP training

GP training initiatives incorporating the Situational Approach are already in place in the UK (with the likelihood of adoption by the NHS in the very near future). These programs can be replicated or used as the basis for further development. Many other GP training initiatives throughout Australia have the potential to complement this work but require revision to ensure the paradigm of illness and drug treatment does not unduly influence practice.

Gender-specific support

Suicide and self-harm are distinguished by a strong gender difference – most suicide deaths are male, most incidents of self-harm are female. To be more effective in reducing both the toll of suicide deaths and the incidence of self-harm, we need to ensure appropriate evidence-based gender competency training for allied health and human services professionals, as well as key people in organisations prepared to assist with preventative mental health and suicide prevention.

In particular, programs designed to engage with men should be built on sound evidence that acknowledges gender difference in key topics, such as dealing with stress. Equally, programs should be careful to not perpetuate unhelpful stereotypes about men, particularly men who may be experiencing psychological or emotional distress.

Labour market reform

Given that the majority of all suicide deaths are people of working age who are not employed, unemployment and re-employment support should become one of the very highest priorities for suicide prevention activity, with a share of available budgets proportionate to the scale of this challenge.

Genuine job creation, coupled with appropriate re-employment support, must become a national priority. We need to enact significant labour market reform. Alongside this, we must ensure the funds are administered transparently so that the benefits genuinely support unemployed and underemployed people, rather than private employment agencies. This is important, as there is detailed analysis to show that our national employment service, jobactive, is ineffective and wasteful of funds directed into that sector, arguably supporting the private job agencies rather than the unemployed and underemployed people it is designed to support. The 2020 report by Simone Casey and Abigail Lewis, *Redesigning Employment Services after COVID-19*, is a useful tool to consider how to improve re-employment and general support for unemployed and underemployed people, and in particular as a genuine upstream suicide prevention activity.[13] Protocols and measures will need to be designed to ensure accountability for any funding directed into the employment sector.

To fully complement any wider labour market reform, we need to also ensure realistic income support until individuals can procure appropriate employment. And we need to offer financial advice and support to unemployed and underemployed people along the way, and to lobby to change the policies of financial institutions to allow more flexibility for those in debt.

Information distribution

The thorough dissemination of appropriate information is fundamental to the transition to more effective suicide prevention efforts. This is a huge task and will require considerable funding; funding that could be re-directed away from the current ineffective approaches, toward information and activities that offer a better chance of reducing our suicide toll.

We need to ensure commonly held beliefs and perceptions are clearly challenged across all levels of our community, and that community-led campaigns offer appropriate messages. A number of high-profile, well-funded campaigns offer ideas and information that are at best ambiguous, and at worst potentially harmful to those in distress.

We need a major integrated information and messaging distribution strategy, with the key content components being wholesale change, appropriate language, new resources, revised and re-analysed data, marketing and distribution strategies, and policy development.

Adopting a new conceptual framework

A major information strategy is needed to promote the Situational Approach as a new and more appropriate conceptual framework, and to explain the extent of the change required to become more effective. This strategy must target all levels of government, the broadest range of sectors, particularly human resources, and throughout the general community.

Appropriate language

As explored earlier, adopting more appropriate language is vital for more effective suicide prevention and effective mental health literacy initiatives that promote the psychological and emotional wellbeing and mental health of individuals and our community. Such language is a vital centrepiece of the Situational Approach. Promoting language and definitions that preserve people's dignity and de-mystify high-intensity mental health difficulties can counter both the conflation of mental illness and suicide, and the conflation of intentional non-fatal self-harm with suicidality. As mentioned, this book provides a language resource to help facilitate this process (see Appendix D: Appropriate language for suicide prevention and the mental health sector).

New resources

We need to design and distribute a new, comprehensive set of resources that cover a range of core topics, such as the Situational Approach, the necessary training, the evidence base (including revised and re-analysed data), and how community activity can become more effective.

Revised and re-analysed data

An integral part of all these activities is the need to thoroughly disseminate revised and re-analysed data (some of which is provided or referenced in this book) – particularly the data around the causes of suicide deaths.

Marketing and distribution strategies

There will need to be comprehensive, well-funded marketing and distribution strategies for information that supports the overall objective of transitioning to a more effective approach to suicide prevention. This will ensure that community activists, employees and volunteers throughout the mental health/suicide prevention sector, human resources personnel, and people throughout the broader community are presented with new, evidence-based information representing a broadly endorsed Situational Approach. To ensure messaging is appropriate, it is crucial that journalists understand their responsibility in providing appropriate information to the community.

Policy development

To enable the implementation of a new Situational Approach to suicide prevention, and because the narrative around mental illness pervades the broadest range of sectors and settings including the HR industry and the workplace generally, all relevant sectors will require an appropriate revision of their mental health policies. We will need strong policy revision throughout the relevant areas of:

- government (federal, state and local)
- industry – particularly human resources

- human services – including welfare, employment, health/mental health and housing
- not-for-profit sector
- philanthropy
- education (all levels) – including:
  - schools
  - coursework and research
  - all mental health/suicide prevention study.

To facilitate this process, those leading the adoption of the new approach will need to consult more broadly with governments, industry (particularly the human resources, training and development, and corporate social responsibility sectors), the health/mental health sector and the human services sectors.

Comprehensive professional development will also be essential to ensure personnel at all levels can meaningfully contribute to the development of new and more appropriate policies.

On the matter of school policies relating to children's mental health; the current practice of large-scale diagnosing of children with mental disorders such as depression, anxiety disorder and the attention deficit disorders is highly questionable and potentially harmful for many children, and there needs to be a thorough revision of all aspects of this process.

Crisis support services

Although many of our crisis support services do a commendable job at the crisis-end of the suicide prevention spectrum, they nevertheless also need to ensure their staff are fully trained and understand their responsibility to move beyond the current thinking as they are an important and integral part of the overall mental health/suicide prevention sector. If they are to work with – and complement – the upstream prevention activity, they need to have a strong sense of the value of the Situational Approach as the conceptual framework for a more effective suicide prevention sector.

Research

We need to develop a new national research policy stating clearly the priorities required to achieve effective suicide prevention; we need to re-prioritise and emphasise the factors known to highly correlate with suicide deaths, such as unemployment, financial hardship, legal and judicial challenges, family breakdown and single status.

We need to simultaneously reduce the emphasis on those aspects of mental health where the demonstrated relationships with suicide are contentious and ambiguous, particularly the focus on depression as causal, and ensure that funding for research is properly overseen, to ensure quality research that aligns with the evidence base and principles of the Situational Approach. This would require:

- effective consultation and re-invigorated leadership in the academic/research domain
- re-alignment of research funding to better explore the evidence base for interventions
- a significant move away from the current Default Depression culture and paradigm of illness in mental health – de-emphasising the identification and diagnosis of mental disorders, particularly depression
- a new approach to data collection – a proposed matrix is outlined below.

Creating a National Data Matrix

The Situational Approach Data Matrix proposes a comprehensive alternative approach to research:

Situational suicide prevention requires a different approach to the use of available suicide data. Adopting a situational suicide prevention model requires a new approach to data collection, integration, and cross-referencing – one that provides a data set encompassing: national, state, and local government areas (and any available individual community data), as well as ranked (where possible) high-risk issues and at-risk sub-groups. This allows for drawing-down visualised data (including with graphs and cross-referenced representations) to inform and guide any one or a combination of different suicide prevention strategies. This facility will provide for the targeting of:

- *particular local government areas and their communities with known high suicide mortality. This provides a basis for identifying and prioritising conspicuous local high-risk issues and at-risk sub-groups, cross referenced with ranked high risk and at-risk sub-group data.*
- *one or more high-risk issues and at-risk sub-groups across the whole population (or a sub-population). However, such a focus still needs to be referenced to data on local government areas (and their communities). An approach to suicide prevention that simply targets known high-risk issues or at-risk subgroups in a general way can be wasteful of resources, and can make it more difficult to evaluate the effectiveness of programs. Focusing prevention efforts generally on subgroups like unemployed or Aboriginal youth, or issues like unemployment or Aboriginal youth suicide, may not be appropriate in communities with little or no suicide mortality history. For example, a community with high unemployment, or a large Indigenous male youth population, may have no history of suicide because of historically effective local support and socio-cultural characteristics that mitigate suicide risk.*
- *events (such as adverse climatic events and industry closure) that are known to escalate suicide risk for certain cohorts, in regions, local government areas, or communities that are affected.*

While we need to innovate and do a better job of bringing together and cross-referencing existing credible sources of data germane to suicide prevention, just as important is admitting what we don't know in order to set a useful new agenda for researchers in this field, and to avoid wasting precious resources on initiatives that are not clearly indicated or justified by available data.[14]

Where to from here?

The current narrative around mental illness – including medicalising common human experience – now pervades every sector of our community. Default Depression – that is, automatically interpreting distress as mental disorder – is central to this.

This has harmful consequences for a great many people, and enormous costs – social and economic – are borne by our community.

There is good evidence that there is substantial over diagnosis of common mental disorders, including depression, anxiety disorder and the attention deficit disorders. Exacerbating this is the concern that treatment for mental disorders is not always suitable to the patients and, in the case of many drugs including antidepressants, may well be harmful.

The current approach and paradigm of illness has widespread influence on government and workplace policy, as well as key industry and community sectors including general practice, the health/mental health sector and human resources. Workplace mental health training is now a huge business in its own right and is a major contributing factor to the spread of key aspects of the current approach, such as interpreting evidence of distress as symptoms of mental disorder. This is Default Depression in action.

Despite enormous funding directed into the mental health/suicide prevention sector, the numbers of suicide deaths continue to rise; and rather than review the general approach, the leadership of this sector continues to promote activities and messages that effectively endorse the key dynamics of the current approach. In particular, the focus on depression remains a core part of the activity of this sector. If we are to begin to reduce the ever-increasing toll of suicide deaths and provide appropriate support for people in distress, we need to enact substantial change to this sector, as a starting point.

Progress will require that well-intentioned and well-informed workers and community activists in the mental health/suicide prevention sector are prepared to:

- challenge public policy
- challenge the direction of funding
- challenge researchers and academics
- call to increase focus on upstream prevention activity to address the major causal factors such as unemployment
- ensure information is accurate and not a distortion of the overall picture
- ensure evidence is not simply cherry-picked to suit the agendas and business interests of those who profit from the current approach.

It is hoped that this book represents the opportunity to channel the heartfelt passion throughout the country to properly address these challenges. In Australia, there are more than enough resources, competent people at all levels and, now, an appropriate conceptual framework – the Situational Approach – with which to lay the foundations for more effective work in the mental health/suicide prevention sector.

Appendix A

Intentional self-harm top 10 multiple causes, proportion of total suicides, by age group, 2017

Cause of death and ICD code	5–24 years	25–44 years	45–64 years	65–84 years	85 years +	All ages
Mood disorders (F30–F39)	34.3	43.0	49.0	40.3	26.0	43.0
Mental and behavioural disorders due to psychoactive substance use (F10–F19)	25.9	41.6	26.7	10.1	2.6	29.5
Other symptoms and signs involving emotional state (R458) (c)	20.6	16.9	19.5	16.4	11.7	18.1
Anxiety and stress-related disorders (F40–F49)	15.2	19.7	17.9	13.6	9.1	17.5
Findings of alcohol, drugs and other substances in blood (R78)	18.5	17.0	13.7	9.6	7.8	14.9
Schizophrenia, schizotypal and delusional disorders (F20–F29)	3.5	7.9	5.2	2.3	—	5.5
Unspecified mental disorder (F99)	7.2	5.0	4.3	1.8	—	4.5
Malignant neoplasms (C00–C97, D45–D46, D47.1, D47.3–D47.5)	0.5	0.9	1.9	16.1	24.7	3.7
Diseases of the musculoskeletal system (M00–M99)	0.2	1.7	3.3	11.1	15.6	3.6
Personality disorders (F60–F69)	5.4	5.0	2.0	1.3	—	3.5
Chronic pain (R522)	0.5	1.3	3.7	5.3	5.2	2.6
Ischaemic heart diseases (I20–I25)	0.2	0.7	1.8	7.8	16.9	2.3
Chronic lower respiratory diseases (J40–J47)	0.2	0.5	2.0	6.0	9.1	1.9
Diabetes (E10–E14)	0.5	0.6	2.0	5.0	9.1	1.8
Heart failure (I50–I51)	0.2	0.2	1.0	5.0	7.8	1.2
Behavioural disorders usually occurring in childhood and adolescence (F90–F98)	3.7	1.1	0.6	—	—	1.1
Disorders of psychological development (F80–F89)	2.1	0.5	0.1	—	—	0.5

* Includes ICD-10 codes X60–X84 and Y87.0. Care needs to be taken in interpreting figures relating to suicide. See Explanatory Notes 91–100.
† Causes of death data for 2017 are preliminary and subject to a revisions process. See Explanatory Notes 57–60.
‡ Includes suicide ideation.
— nil or rounded to zero (including null cells)
From Australian Bureau of Statistics, '3303.0 - Causes of Death, Australia, 2017', published 26 September 2018, https://www.abs.gov.au/ausstats/abs@.nsf/Lookup/by%20Subject/3303.0~2017~Main%20Features~Intentional%20 self-harm,%20key%20characteristics~3.

Appendix B

National Coronial Information System

DR16-16: Intentional Self-Harm Fatalities in Australia, 2001–2013

Table 1. Intentional Self-Harm Fatalities in Australia by Employment Status and Age Range

Age Range [Year]	Employed	Unemployed	Retired Pensioner	Unlikely to be known	Student	Home Duties	Prisoner	Other	Child not at school	Total
15–19	395	384	13	114	590	4	6	1	2	1509
20–24	1071	783	52	296	315	27	25	6	0	2575
25–29	1347	940	87	339	110	51	24	3	0	2901
30–34	1564	949	190	377	61	79	34	4	0	3258
35–39	1671	920	239	396	48	85	29	3	0	3391
40–44	1722	853	294	407	26	83	20	4	0	3409
45–49	1614	753	330	351	11	72	10	7	0	3148
50–54	1266	562	451	312	10	67	7	4	0	2679
55–59	848	393	528	218	6	74	4	6	0	2077
60–65	539	150	923	164	0	44	8	4	0	1832
Total	**12,037**	**6687**	**3107**	**2974**	**1177**	**586**	**167**	**42**	**2**	**26,779**

From Eva Saar and Thomas Burgess, 'Intentional Self-Harm Fatalities in Australia 2001–2013. Data Report DR16 – 16 (2016) National Coronial Information System', http://malesuicidepreventionaustralia.com.au/wp-content/uploads/2017/01/NCIS-Report-2016_FINAL.pdf.

Appendix C

Proportion of workers' compensation claims involving a 'mental condition', 2015

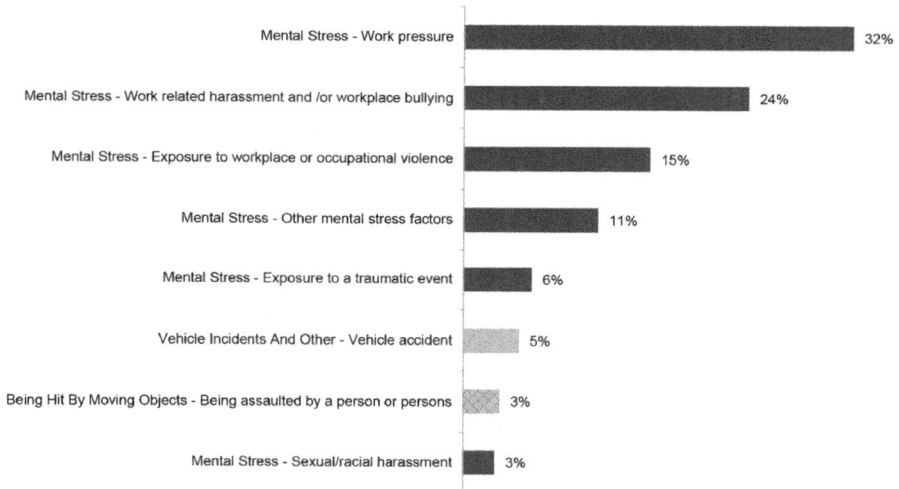

From Safe Work Australia, *Work Related Mental Disorders Profile (2015)* https://www.safeworkaustralia.gov.au/system/files/documents/1702/work-related-mental-disorders-profile.pdf

Appendix D

Appropriate language for suicide prevention
and the mental health sector

Choosing language that helps rather than harms

The use of appropriate language is crucial to facilitating appropriate care and support for people in distress. Pathologising language, using words such as 'disorder' and 'illness', and particularly diagnostic labels such as 'depression' and 'anxiety disorder', are far from innocuous. In fact, they can be harmful. Such language can be derogatory, and can contribute to stigma and social marginalisation. It can also transform the way people see and define themselves, often for a lifetime. In particular, it can disempower people, making them feel helpless and reliant on expert intervention. Providing a succinct, non-clinical description with appropriate language may be reassuring, with less risk of adverse negative effects.

This document is part language guide, part glossary. It discusses language that is useful and language that is problematic, to provide guidance to health/welfare practitioners, and concerned members of the community. It provides a practical set of terms and definitions for dealing with the distress related to a broad spectrum of human difficulties experienced by many people and frequently encountered by practitioners in the suicide prevention/mental health field.

The Situational Approach is a new conceptual framework for how we consider and respond to human distress. It focuses on situational distress rather than mental disorders. It is underpinned by recognition of the need to acknowledge and address wider issues that are contributing to distress (including unemployment, poverty, relationship problems, and grief). It has been developed to encourage appropriate, competent, caring responses to individuals in distress.

The Situational Approach is a significant departure from the current medical framework for suicide prevention and mental health, with its emphasis on illness and the use of pathologising language relating to mental health.

This appropriate language guide is a companion to the book *Default Depression – How we now interpret distress as mental illness.*

Appropriate terminology

The terms and language below draw on a variety of sources. The definitions are not meant to be considered as exhaustive or final and are likely to evolve and be refined as the Situational Approach becomes more firmly established as a suitable conceptual framework for the mental health/suicide prevention sector. Some of the terms below are new and come from the Situational Approach. Others are already in common usage, but are clarified here to facilitate a more appropriate and less-medicalised approach to dealing with distress.

Table 1. Key terms

situational distress	**Situational distress** encompasses a significantly challenging or troubling experience of thoughts, emotions, bodily sensations, or behaviours, associated with difficult life events, such as bereavement, a change in health status, relationship breakdown, financial, or occupational difficulties. This distress may significantly overlap with many of the symptoms usually taken to suggest mental disorders (such as depression and anxiety).[1]
	The conceptual basis for situational distress acknowledges social determinants such as unemployment, and financial and relationship difficulties, as having a key role as causal factors in distress. However, sometimes in cases of acute distress, there are no evident social causal factors, such as with some high-intensity mental health difficulties like schizophrenic or other psychotic experiences. Notwithstanding, the situational context remains a vitally important consideration. In the case of suicidality and death by suicide, the situational context is also a vital consideration.
	Regardless of the causal factors involved, people in extreme distress need their situational context – including family context, finances, health/mental health and community support services availability – to be considered as a priority for appropriate responses and ongoing care and support.

psychological distress	**Psychological distress** refers to patterns of psychological and emotional discomfort and general unpleasant feelings and emotions. It is an umbrella term to describe some common interrelated identifiable patterns of difficulty including stress, insomnia, depression, anxiety and suicidal thoughts. Psychological distress may be associated with factors such as: interpersonal difficulties, bereavement, lack of sleep, use of drugs or alcohol, workplace stress or abuse and physical illness. Some of the most potent factors associated with psychological distress are thoughts and feelings of powerlessness. For distressed individuals, feeling powerless, and perceiving themselves to be powerless, can result in a decline in general mental capacity (thinking, problem solving, and memory recall), irritability, anger, and diminished verbal communication.[2] The stress of this experience can trigger multi-system changes in the body,[3] further compounding the difficulties an individual may face. Although people suffering psychological distress may experience a great deal of difficulty in their general mental capacity, this should not be presumed to be a psychiatric disorder or illness.
high-intensity psychological distress	**High-intensity psychological distress** refers to acute psychological and emotional distress which may require direct supportive intervention. People suffering high intensity psychological distress may be at elevated risk of suicide.[4] This level of distress usually significantly impairs a person's ability to function on a day-to-day basis and noticeably interferes with their usual or preferred mental, emotional, or social capacity, and their experience of feeling capable and competent. Distress of this intensity often requires more than a person's own coping ability, lifestyle adjustments, and support of friends and family. At least initially, it may require thoughtful observation and reflective assessment by a qualified health professional (a doctor, psychotherapist, psychologist, or, in some cases, a psychiatrist), who may also suggest appropriate psychotherapy (psychological therapy). It is important to understand that having experiences such as schizophrenia or psychotic episodes does not necessarily make a person suicidal, and that, with the right support, people who have these experiences can live a satisfactory and manageable life.[5] In this regard, the World Health Organization (WHO) emphasises psychosocial interventions as particularly important support strategies.[6] The term 'high intensity psychological distress' is proposed as a less pathologising alternative to the commonly used but restrictive and ambiguous terms such as mental disorder or mental illness.

suicidality	**Suicidality** refers to a range of states from suicidal ideation (having serious thoughts about suicide and taking one's own life), through planning a suicide death and on through to attempted suicide. It is quite common for people to have serious thoughts about taking their own life – in 2020–2021, 1 in 6 (16.7% or around 3.3 million) of Australians aged 16–85 had serious thoughts about taking their own life at some point in their lives.[7] People who experience all forms of suicidal thoughts and behaviours (suicidality) are at greater risk of completing suicide.[8] However, it is important to understand that although people who experience suicidal ideation and even make suicide plans are at increased risk of further suicide attempts, most do not go on to kill themselves.
	There is a gender-based paradox to suicidality; despite the much higher rate of completed male suicides, females are more likely to be suicidal than males, with significantly higher rates of suicidal ideation (2.7% versus 1.9%), and suicide plans and (incomplete) attempts.[9] This disparity can be explained to some extent at least by understanding the different physiological reactions including the different primary role hormones play for males and females when under stress.[10]
self-harm	**Self-harm** refers to deliberate self-injury or other physical harm such as cutting, burning, poisoning, or overdosing on drugs (including prescription medications) and/or alcohol.
	Self-harm is common, and not only among teenagers.[11] However, it is crucial to note that, in most cases, self-harm is not an attempt at suicide and does not lead to suicide.[12]
	The relationship between suicide and self-harm is complicated. People with a history of self-harm are at considerably higher risk of suicide.[13] However, there is some evidence, including a Finnish study[14] and an American study,[15] that many, perhaps the majority, of suicide deaths occur on the first attempt.
	Although there is some overlap between people who attempt but do not complete suicide and those who do complete suicide, these groups are characterised by significant demographic and clinical differences.[16]
	Most cases of self-harm occur in females, as do most cases of attempted but incomplete suicide; but most suicide deaths occur in males.[17] In many cases of self-harm, there is a history of behavioural difficulties, substance misuse, and family, social, and psychological problems.[18] None of this should be automatically presumed to indicate a mental disorder.
	Self-harm should always be taken seriously, whether or not the intention is suicide.

There is a situational context relevant to every suicide death. Very often, there is substantial situational distress in the preceding days, weeks, months, or even years.

Extensive research shows that many people who kill themselves have no history of mental disorder and/or are impacted by difficult social circumstances.[19] The majority of people who kill themselves have been in circumstances likely to cause enormous stress in their lives, such as unemployment – the majority of all suicide deaths in Australia are people of working age who were not employed at the time of their death.[20] It is crucial that this issue be considered as a priority in current and future suicide prevention planning and initiatives.

People suffering high intensity psychological distress (see definition above) may be at elevated risk of suicide. This distress is often associated with difficult social and financial circumstances which may precipitate a state of despair or hopelessness. Such people may be greatly in need of and may benefit from timely and competent professional support. Regardless of the associated factors, it may further compound the difficulties being faced by people in distress to reduce the scope of support solely to health/mental health professionals.

Many people who die by suicide have recently engaged with a mental health professional.[21] Limiting preventive strategies to those built upon the presumption of mental disorder or illness will simply not help many, perhaps the majority, of people at risk of suicide. There is also evidence showing that inappropriate support can discourage people away from seeking help again.[22] Effective suicide prevention requires that measures of prevention are non-pathologising, informed by evidence-based, gender-specific differences in help seeking, and part of a broader, more encompassing approach that takes account of social determinants.

Risk factors and protective factors

Suicide prevention activity should be informed by known risk factors and protective factors. There are many known risk factors associated with stress in a person's life that may contribute/lead to suicide. It is important for effective suicide prevention that we design and target prevention activities according to the prevalence and strength of the risk factors in different demographic groups.

Risk and protective factors for psychological or emotional wellbeing act at several different levels, consequently responses to these factors need to be multi-layered and multi-sectoral. Health, education, welfare, transport, and housing sectors are all crucially important and need to be involved at the core of any preventive activity. It is important that these key agencies outside health/mental health have a vital leadership role in suicide prevention rather than just as a superficial 'partner' to health/mental health in order to fulfil token inter-agency requirements.

Table 2. Risk factors and protective factors

at-risk	In general, **at-risk** refers to individuals and groups who have higher rates of suicide compared with the general population. Identifying people at-risk can play an important role in helping focus preventive activities.
risk factors	**Risk factors** are factors that may negatively impact on a person's life and experience in a way that potentially increases the likelihood of suicide. Key risk factors for suicide include social determinants such as unemployment, financial difficulties and homelessness, as well as high intensity psychological difficulties (such as some psychiatric conditions), prior suicide attempts, alcohol misuse, serious health challenges, childhood abuse, psychological trauma, grief, separation and divorce, and the experience of powerlessness. Risk factors vary relative to age, gender, and other intersecting social and cultural factors. However, the evidence suggests that in many, and perhaps the majority of cases, multiple risk factors combine to elevate psychological distress to intolerable levels. Several risk factors may be influential at multiple levels and may overlap.[23]
proximal risk factors	**Proximal risk** factors are those that have a more direct and immediate influence on a person's level of psychological distress. These may exacerbate existing life challenges. Proximal risk factors are similar to adverse life events – examples include the failure of a person's business, a farmer's experience of prolonged drought, unemployment, relationship breakdown and serious health issues.[24]

acute intervention	**Acute intervention** refers to engagement by health/welfare workers with individuals who are already so highly psychologically distressed they are at a greater risk of self-harm or suicide.
	Ideally, acute intervention would occur in broader settings than just the medical/ mental health domain, and should include all relevant government agencies (such as housing and employment support) as well as not-for-profit and community care organisations.
	It is important at the individual level, but it has limited preventive impact at the population level.[36]
crisis intervention	Like acute intervention, **crisis intervention** refers to engaging directly with individuals who are at high risk of imminent self-harm or suicide.
suicide postvention	**Suicide postvention** refers to follow-up support for people affected by a suicide death or incomplete attempted suicide. Suicide postvention may include grief counselling and preventive support for family and friends of individuals who have died by suicide.
	This support is vitally important, because family and friends may be at increased risk of suicide themselves, because of their responses to the suicide (e.g. grief and/or guilt). However, like any other later intervention, postvention is limited in its scope of prevention, because it generally only targets people who have been identified by health/support services as being at-risk through their connection to individual suicide deaths or incomplete suicide attempts.

Problematic terms and concepts

The effectiveness of research and practice in the mental health/suicide prevention sector has been hindered by ambiguity and unhelpful terminology. It is important for effective work in this sector that key terms and concepts are used appropriately. Despite the good intentions of many people working in the suicide prevention/mental health sectors, some of the terminology in common usage appears to be misunderstood or misused.

distal risk factors	Distal risk factors are historical and contextual factors that may put someone at later risk of suicide; such factors predispose a person to an inherent vulnerability. Examples of distal risk factors include childhood abuse or other trauma such as sustained poverty, poor social service support and the trauma experienced by returned veterans.[25]
protective factors	Protective factors are those aspects of a person's life that make it less likely that they will die by suicide. They mitigate or lessen the risk of suicide. Protective factors may be present in all aspects of a person's life, throughout the lifespan. Examples of key protective factors for people in distress may include proactive interpersonal and social support of family, friends, and/or work colleagues, and constructive help-seeking. Work can be a protective factor, above and beyond the financial benefits, providing social interaction/support, meaningful activity, and engendering self-esteem. Other protective factors include policies and practices that restrict means of suicide.[26] Effective, humane institutional and service/agency support is also protective. At the broader social level, protective factors need to be articulated and enshrined in social policy that addresses the social determinants of health and wellbeing. Protective factors are related to resilience, and both have individual and social dimensions; individuals can be more resilient in the face of adversity where there are good social support structures in place.
social determinants	Social determinants of physical and mental health are social, economic, and material factors, including income, employment status, working conditions, education, housing, food security, transport, and social inclusion/(non) discrimination. Social determinants of mental health profoundly affect mental health, and are an appropriate focus for population-level mental health promotion. The acronyms 'SDOH' and 'SDH' are often used for social determinants of health. We use 'SDOMH' for social determinants of mental health. The situational approach to suicide prevention and mental health has much in common with a SDOMH perspective, but it is more directly applicable at an individual/clinical level, as well as being relevant to population-level interventions.

structural determinants	**Structural determinants** are root causes of health disparities, including political/economic/ social policies, and regulatory and administrative processes, that affect income, working conditions, housing, and education, etc.
	Structural determinants overlap with social determinants, but the term more specifically refers to political and economic factors.
biopsychosocial factors	**Biopsychosocial factors** are a broad range of factors with potential to impact on an individual's wellbeing; an individual's health and wellbeing is influenced by their biology, and by psychological and social factors. The idea of interacting systems at both the individual and social levels is a core concept of the biopsychosocial model. Even intense 'inner' psychological distress must be seen as part of a broader set of influences. Any resolution of this distress can only be achieved by acknowledging and working with these interactive factors[27].
adverse (negative) life events	Nearly all suicides appear to be associated with at least one (usually more) **adverse life event** within one year of death, and this is concentrated in the last few months prior to death.[28]
	The international literature on risk factors for suicide consistently identifies a range of adverse life events and stressful challenges associated with suicide. Precipitating events have been found in up to 96% of suicides, with studies showing that social factors play a key role in suicide risk.[29]
	Adverse life events may include unemployment, relationship breakdown, collapse of an individual's business, a farmer's experience of prolonged drought, and serious health issues, illness or death of a family member. Often there is no single adverse event but rather the accumulation of a series of adverse life events that combine to lead to what is described in published research as 'pathways to despair' and suicide death.[30]

The spectrum of suicide prevention activity

Currently, suicide prevention initiatives occur across a broad spectrum of activity representing two broadly different orientations and approaches (Figure 1), which need to be better integrated. The different models can generally be broken down into: (1) a broadscale, population-wide strategies, and (2) more targeted strategies such as support for individuals who are acutely distressed and at-risk, and follow-up support for people bereaved by suicide and people who have non-fatally self-harmed.

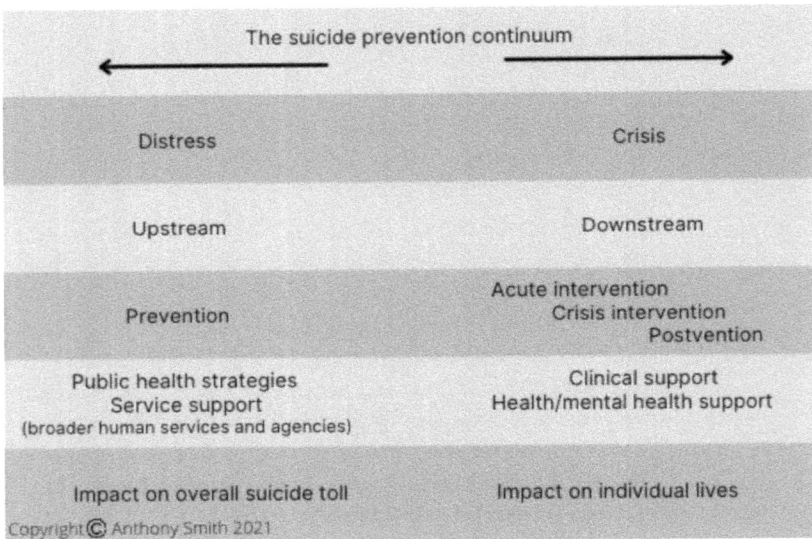

Figure 1. The suicide prevention spectrum

There are different levels of prevention. Much of the current approach to suicide prevention sits within the downstream, acute level of intervention. Although important in responding to people identified as being of elevated risk of suicide, this level of intervention fails to alter the trajectory of escalating risk for many people who go on to kill themselves. Such interventions cannot be expected to reduce the overall toll of suicide deaths. The limited impact of downstream interventions on the overall suicide toll is further compounded by ineffectual upstream interventions that are influenced by mental illness ideology, for example the promotion of depression screening, despite evidence that it is ineffective and may be harmful.[31]

Health and human service agency responses to suicide in Australia are generally known by the generic term 'suicide prevention'. However, much of the work done in this field, although vitally important, is not so much preventive as a reactive response to the tragedy of suicide. Although reactive interventions have an important preventive role – such as providing follow-up support for people personally affected by suicide – they have limited preventive impact at the population level.[32]

Effective suicide prevention requires that all levels of intervention be evidence-based and subjected to rigorous evaluation.[33]

Table 3. Prevention levels and strategies

upstream prevention	**Upstream prevention** addresses financial, environmental, industrial and economic structures and conditions that may impact negatively on the wellbeing of individuals in the overall population or population subgroups.
	Effective upstream prevention activity is required to reduce the overall toll of suicide deaths. To be effective, upstream prevention activity should address fundamental social and economic structures that can enable improved social support and general protective factors across the total population. This can be done through appropriate broadscale public health and health promotion activity, in which health professionals can take an advocacy role in interagency work with key government departments and activity such as housing and infrastructure.
	This level or type of activity is distinct from the later, intervention and postvention (or downstream prevention), activity which tends to focus on individuals. Common current upstream prevention activities include public awareness campaigns, community outreach services, and community education.
	Key factors in suicide deaths such as unemployment, financial difficulties, and housing insecurity often cause intense distress. Appropriate population-level interventions to support people experiencing these challenges should primarily focus on activity outside the health/mental health sector, such as job-creation, re-employment support, housing affordability policies, and financial support programs.

downstream prevention	Downstream prevention refers to activity that is generally limited to dealing directly with individuals who have been identified as at-risk of suicide, and/or ongoing postvention support (e.g. counselling/psychotherapy) for family and friends affected by suicide and suicidality.
	Although downstream prevention is vitally important in caring for highly distressed individuals, it cannot play a major role in reducing the overall toll of suicide deaths. This is in large part because many people who die by suicide do not have meaningful engagement, if any engagement at all, with health/support services prior to their death.
public health interventions	**Public health interventions** are population-wide approaches by the health sector, often in collaboration with other sectors, including housing, employment, education, and transport.
	Appropriate public health activity built on good research and planning represents an important opportunity to effectively address the suicide death toll. However, public health activity in the mental health/suicide prevention sector (and the health sector more broadly) has tended to reflect a narrow focus on a medicalised approach, and where there have been attempts to advocate to broaden the focus to include social determinants such as poverty and housing, there has generally not been the political will to enact this in any substantial way.[34]
universal prevention strategies[35]	**Universal prevention strategies** address an entire population (e.g. all residents of a state or country) or cohort (e.g. all primary school students), not just people considered to be at risk. They include programs such as public education campaigns, means restriction, education programs for the media on reporting practices related to suicide, and crisis response plans.
selective prevention strategies	**Selective prevention strategies** address subsets of the total population, focusing on at-risk groups that have a greater probability of becoming suicidal, and are designed to prevent the onset of suicidal behaviours among specific subpopulations. This level of prevention includes screening programs and training for frontline caregivers and peer support workers.
indicated prevention strategies	**Indicated strategies** address specific high-risk individuals within the population – people showing signs of personal crisis and a high risk of suicide.

Table 4. Clarification of some key terms and concepts

rates versus numbers	Both rates and numbers of suicide deaths are important for consideration of appropriate suicide prevention activity. However, either considered alone without reference to the other can give a distorted representation of suicide deaths.
	Rates of suicide are generally measured as deaths per 100,000 of a population group.[37] However, although this facilitates comparisons between different groups, it can give rise to a skewed representation when working with relatively small populations such as in rural areas in Australia. High rates in a small population may justify specific targeted interventions, but this may not lead to a reduction in the overall toll if larger populations with larger numbers of suicide deaths but lower rates are not properly targeted as well.
	Numbers are simply the total numbers of deaths in an area or group. For larger population areas, relatively large numbers of suicide deaths may be reported/ expressed as a relatively lower rate and consequently not receive the attention they deserve.
gender specificity in suicide prevention	The suicide death/self-harm spectrum is strongly gender-specific. Although there is some overlap, the large majority (about 75%) of suicide deaths occur in males, but the large majority of incidents of non-fatal self-harm occur in females.[38] To develop effective preventive activity on this suicide/self-harm spectrum requires clearly defined, evidence-based gender-specific activity on a scale proportionate to the risk level of the target group.
rural versus metropolitan suicide rates	In general, rural rates of suicide are higher than in metropolitan areas. However, the great majority of Australian suicide deaths occur in city-dwelling adults.[39] This is not a contradiction: there are high rates of suicide in many rural areas of Australia, and the development of appropriate preventive activity is required to address this. And although rural rates of suicide are generally higher than metropolitan rates, this is a considerable generalisation: rates vary enormously if measured by locality (for example, local government areas or federal electorates) in both rural and metropolitan areas.[40] Some metropolitan areas have both higher rates of suicide than many rural areas and considerably higher numbers of suicide deaths than many rural areas. The five capital cities of Sydney, Melbourne, Brisbane, Adelaide and Perth together account for over half (54.18%) of all suicide deaths in Australia. Suicide rates tend to be higher in socially and economically disadvantaged areas.[41]
	Note: Torrens University Australia hosts a very good online suicide mapping tool: Torrens University Australia Public Health Information Development Unit (PHIDU) Social Health Atlases. The website hosts interactive maps on health data, including suicide, in multiple geographical areas.

groups with high rates of suicide	As well as high rates of suicide in some rural areas and socially and economically disadvantaged metropolitan areas, there are high rates of suicide among other groups including among Aboriginal people, with very high rates among young Aboriginal males.[42] There are disproportionately high rates of suicide (and attempted suicide) among unemployed people. The majority of all suicide deaths occur in people who are not employed, and there are also high rates of suicide among mature-age men and unemployed people (both male and female).[43, 44] Suicide deaths among people who are not employed account for at least 55% of all suicide deaths of people of working age. For women of working age, there is also a high proportion of suicide deaths among those who are not employed – 68.2%.
youth suicide	When youth suicide is discussed, 'youth' can refer to various age groups, and people often equate 'youth' with 'teenage'. It is important to distinguish between the 15–19 year-old age group and the 15–24 year-old age group, because there are much larger numbers of suicide deaths in 20–24 year olds than in 15–19 year olds (older teenagers).[45] Adding the two age groups together significantly inflates the 'youth' numbers. These inflated figures are then used to argue for program and research funding that largely targets teenagers, while very little suicide prevention activity targets the 20–24 age group.
data collection, analysis, and reporting	Rigorous data gathering and analysis, and reporting evidence with integrity, are vital for effective suicide prevention. Evidence that is viewed from a limited perspective, such as the presumption of widespread mental disorder, based on inflated rates of over-diagnosed depression and anxiety disorders, can be misleading. In Australia, the Australian Bureau of Statistics presents data on causes of death, including suicide. However, the causes of suicide presented are dominated by diagnostic categories such as mental disorders and substance abuse disorders, while important social determinants such as housing difficulties are largely disregarded.[46]

appropriate research methodology	The growing criticism of the current approach to suicide prevention includes fundamental challenges to how we research this subject:
	To date, research has been insufficient to explain why men, especially during middle age, are particularly vulnerable to taking their own lives. The shortcomings of prior studies include lack of longitudinal follow-up, failure to measure such factors as social integration and dimensional indicators of stress, overreliance on categorical measures of psychopathology, and a focus on proxy outcomes instead of death by suicide.[47]
	Suicide prevention research tends to be dominated by a focus on mental illness, particularly depression, and assumptions such as the importance of screening for mental disorders and providing clinical treatment. Although it is important to engage with people who are at risk of suicide and who have already come to the attention of health services, clinical research offers little opportunity for guidance in moving towards more effective population-wide preventive activity.
evidence and evidence base	It is vital that suicide prevention activities are underpinned by robust evidence. As there is a range of different target groups that require different considerations for effective prevention work, properly defining a target group, and suitable prevention activity is fundamental.[48]
	Much of the current approach to suicide prevention appears to be at odds with a good deal of the available evidence, and disregards criticism. It is often too generic and reductionist to be effective. It lacks crucial gender differentiation, frames suicide within a narrow mental disorder paradigm, and tends to ignore compelling recent international research highlighting important social determinants of suicide, such as unemployment.[49]

mental health ideology	The term 'ideology' refers to systematically related beliefs and assumptions that form the basis of a more-or-less coherent perspective. Mental health ideology refers to the broader set of beliefs justifying an over-medicalised approach to distress and other common human behaviours. The general narrative about mental health is founded on a biomedical model – that distress is symptomatic of a mental disorder. In this model, people become patients with psychiatric pathology that is treatable by medical means, often potentially harmful antidepressant drugs.[50] Key aspects of this model include categorising behaviours and psychological/emotional distress as mental disorders, and applying formal medical diagnoses – labelling people as having a mental illness. Using clinical terminology such as 'symptom', 'illness', and 'treatment' in relation to people in distress helps to establish and maintain mental illness ideology. It also helps to legitimise the over-medicalised approach, and influences people to accept it as valid and authoritative. Although the term 'mental health ideology' may be deemed as confrontational, understanding the influence of ideology is important to help counter the prevailing narrative that tends to reduce complex human experiences and feelings to categories of mental disorder.
medicalisation	A key part of the biomedical model is the concept of medicalisation. To medicalise is to reduce and simplify issues of personal health and wellbeing to medical diagnoses, often presuming the need for medical treatment. For suicide prevention, this refers to the process of reducing complex issues of psychological or emotional distress, regardless of the causes of that distress, to medical diagnoses such as depression or anxiety disorder. This is usually followed by treatment, commonly including prescription of potentially harmful pharmaceuticals such as antidepressants (for depression and anxiety disorders) and amphetamine derivatives (for children's behavioural issues).[51] This is not to suggest that appropriate medical intervention is never warranted; but such intervention should always be integrated with a broader contextual, situational approach to care and support.
pathologisation	To pathologise is similar to medicalise – to describe a common human experience as a medical abnormality, disorder or illness; as wrong; as inappropriate. This is all too common in the suicide prevention sector, where the symptoms of stress, or more broadly, psychological distress, are presumed to be evidence of a mental disorder.

workplace mental health	Workplace mental health (WMH) has become a major workplace issue. However, there is international concern about increasing numbers of workers on sickness and disability benefits, with mental disorders disproportionately increasing.[52, 53] In Australia, work-related mental health conditions are now the second most common cause of workers' compensation claims.[54] Regardless of the factors causing workplace stress or trauma, many WMH policies and practices for dealing with worker distress give workers little option but to accept a medicalised pathway and the diagnosis of a mental disorder if they wish to receive ongoing workplace accommodations and/or financial support.[55, 56]
	WMH claims are made to support distressed workers. However, typical insurance industry literature, such as the following from MLC Insurance, advises distressed workers to engage with a GP *as the first step*:
	There are a number of tactics to manage anxiety and depression, including counselling and medication. The first thing to do, however, is to seek help from your doctor, who can then advise on the best course of action.
	A typical part of this process is developing a Mental Health Treatment Plan, with the presumption that clinical depression or anxiety disorder is fundamental to the problem.[57]
	Despite the efforts and enormous funding to 'destigmatise' and the encouragement and messaging for people to 'talk to someone about your mental health', recent data shows that more than half (53%) of Australian workers would hide a mental or physical health condition they had so that they would not be judged or discriminated against.[58, 59] The lack of effectiveness of destigmatisation efforts has led one high profile leader in the mental health arena to openly recommend people not disclose their 'mental illness' to an employer.[60]
workplace mental health training	Workplace mental health training has become an enormous business[61] and most employers are obliged to provide such training. However, much of the training is built around diagnostic labels and other clinical terminology.[62] There is relatively little focus on workplace conditions (e.g. long hours, shift work, lack of job control) or stressful workplace events (e.g. harassment, bullying, violence), or social determinants such as poverty and housing insecurity.

the 'talk to someone' message	The 'talk to someone' message as a preventive strategy is prevalent and has attracted substantial financial backing in mental health campaigns.[63] However, the evidence for the value of this as a population-wide preventive activity is questionable. The occasional anecdotal story of a distressed person who talked to someone, although a favourite with the media, does not constitute evidence or a representative sample supporting the efficacy of this approach. Published research offers a contrasting view altogether; with very recent research showing that this sort of strategy leads a significant proportion of people (especially men) into a very problematic and possibly tragic pathway.[64]
	Rather than a focus on 'talk' as a response to suicide among men, suicide prevention initiatives might instead seek to engage more broadly with economic and housing security, access to non-stigmatizing welfare/disability support, robust programs promoting gender equality, easy access to well-resourced community-based services in relation to mental health and substance use.[65]
	There are important questions to ask about the 'talk to someone' message. Who should people speak with if they are in crisis? What are the appropriate skills for supportive engagement of people whose distress is clearly related to adverse life events? Research has shown that this particular approach may be particularly unhelpful for some men:
	It may be the case that common suicide prevention strategies, such as encouraging greater use of mental health services by men and focusing on raising awareness of links between mental illness and suicide, are unlikely to lead to effective interventions for such individuals.[66]

To facilitate more appropriate language use, this section discusses some of the more problematic terms in common usage, and offers some options for alternative language.

Table 5. Problematic terms

Terms to consider avoiding unless properly clarified	Recommended terms/language
depression – highly ambiguous; confuses and conflates normal (albeit sometimes distressing and highly challenging) human experience with pathological categorisations; perpetuates medicalisation/pathologisation; questionable taxonomic integrity.	Distress, psychological/emotional distress. When relevant, call it what it actually is – for example, emotional difficulty, mood disturbance, melancholy, negative introspection, loneliness or grief.
anxiety disorder – can be ambiguous; tends to disregard situational stress (which is not the same as anxiety except in some features of physiology).	Anxiety.
mental illness/mental disorder – as with *depression*, both terms are highly ambiguous; perpetuate medicalisation/pathologisation; questionable taxonomic integrity.	For the purposes of effective suicide prevention, it is better to avoid these terms altogether, if possible, or at least to provide a clarification of the context and meaning of the terms as they are used.
mental health – so highly ambiguous as to seriously restrict the understanding of the broader context and factors involved in an individual's distress; implies an opposite – that is, mental ill-health/mental disorder; serves to endorse the medicalisation of distress and limit the scope of interventions and prevention to experts in the mental health field. 'Mental health' is often used as a euphemism for mental illness.	Wellbeing; health and wellbeing; personal/psychological/emotional wellbeing. Social and emotional wellbeing (SEWB) – a term commonly used by Aboriginal and Torres Strait Islander people (Indigenous Australians).[67]
mental health expert	Describe by relevant occupation – for example, psychologist, psychiatrist, mental health nurse, or researcher.
'living with' a mental disorder – a very commonly used term. It is considered respectful, but it is problematic. In particular, it implies chronicity. It also implies that mental disorders dominate and define people, eclipsing other aspects of their lives. It can be inadvertently disempowering and patronising.	Experiencing distress. Diagnosed with a mental disorder.

mental health literacy – a commonly used term, but it is problematic. It encourages people to interpret their experience, and other people's experience, particularly distress, through a mental health/illness lens, and it rarely if ever includes a consideration of SDOMH.	
resilience – this should be the concept of resilience that has become a favourite in mental health literature and training. Unfortunately, it is often used in a way that largely focuses responsibility on individuals to rely on personal resources/attributes to weather difficult times, deflecting attention from the social/economic/political factors that contribute to hardship.[68]	

Depression and anxiety

Despite many suicides deaths having no evidence of prior mental disorder, and the strong place of adverse life events in suicide deaths, much of the current approach continues to push the paradigm of illness and mental deficiency and the unhelpful focus on categories of mental disorder.

Table 6. Depression and anxiety

depression	There is an enormous body of published literature questioning not just the role of depression in suicide deaths but also key aspects of the conceptualisation of depression. The experience of being human can sometimes be acutely distressing, even overwhelming and debilitating. Nevertheless, such experience does not necessarily constitute a diagnosable mental illness, and in fact is often a normal response to stressful events such as financial difficulties, workplace problems, or housing problems.
anxiety disorder	Anxiety is a perfectly natural human experience. It is a reaction to stress that has both psychological and physical features. Some experts consider that stress, anxiety, and depression are different aspects of the same psychological distress, and that making a distinction between anxiety and depression is unhelpful.[69] Anxiety levels for some people may become overwhelming and chronic, with a debilitating impact on their daily lives, and they may need treatment. However, anxiety should not be automatically presumed to be a mental disorder. Causes of the stress should always be considered in supporting people with anxiety.

Further reading

This appropriate language guide is a companion to the book *Default Depression – How we now interpret distress as mental illness.*

Acknowledgements

A number of people have generously supported and encouraged me along the way in preparing this book. Some of the support has been from friends, some who already supported the general thrust of the book and some who have been impacted in one way or another by aspects of some of the difficulties described in the book.

I would especially like to thank and acknowledge:

John Ashfield, for putting in the time and effort into the first Situational Approach papers; and in particular for developing some of the definitions in those papers that are a key part of the Stand-Alone. John Macdonald, for reading an early draft and encouraging me all the while through the long times of re-workings. Melissa Raven, especially for her considerable time and patience in helping with the editing and revising of the Stand-Alone. Steph Lightfoot did the initial editing prior to submission; Steph did a great job, was easy to work with and her enthusiasm for the general content and analysis, some of it new to her, was very heartening for me.

Others read early drafts and gave valuable feedback and support, in particular Bill Power and Virginia Swanton, my cousin Helene Powell and Elizabeth Webb.

It has been a good experience to work on this project with Wakefield Press, in particular Julia Beaven, as editor, has contributed significantly, over and above her general editing role. She has a strong background and understanding of many of the key issues in the book and in many cases throughout the editing process she has enabled the better articulation of important points.

Notes

Preface

1   Read, J., 2007, 'Why promoting biological ideology increases prejudice against people labelled "schizophrenic"' in *Australian Psychologist* 42, no. 2: 118–128, https://doi.org/10.1080/00050060701280607

2   Australian Bureau of Statistics (ABS), 2016, *3303.0 – Causes of Death, Australia, 2015* published 28 September 2016, https://www.abs.gov.au/AUSSTATS/abs@.nsf/Details Page/3303.02015?OpenDocument; Australian Bureau of Statistics. *Causes of Death, Australia* (Belconnen, ACT: ABS, 2020), https://www.abs.gov.au/statistics/health/causes-death/causes-death-australia/latest-release#data-download

3   Safe Work Australia, 'Mental Health', https://www.safeworkaustralia.gov.au/topic/mental-health; Mazza, D., Brijnath, B., Chakraborty, S.P. and the Guideline Development Group. 2019, 'Clinical guideline for the diagnosis and management of work-related mental health conditions in general practice'. Melbourne: Monash Universityhttps://www.racgp.org.au/clinical-resources/clinical-guidelines/guidelines-by-topic/mental-health-1/diagnosis-and-management-of-work-related-mental-he; Harvey, S.B., Joyce, S., Modini, M., et al., 'Work and depression/anxiety disorders – a systematic review of reviews' (Beyond Blue, 2012), https://www.beyondblue.org.au/about-us/research-projects/research-projects/work-and-depression-anxiety-disorders-a-systematic-review-of-reviews; WorkSafe Victoria, *Mental Injury Support*, Melbourne: State of Victoria, 2020, https://www.worksafe.vic.gov.au/mental-injury-support

4   The Royal Australian College of General Practitioners, 2018, *General Practice: Health of the Nation 2018* (East Melbourne, Victoria: 2018, https://www.racgp.org.au/getmedia/b123611e-e423-4bc8-8665-949e4bed9792/Health-of-the-Nation-2018-report.pdf.aspx

5   Baldwin, M., and Marcus, S., 2007, 'Labor Market Outcomes of Persons with Mental Disorders' in *Industrial Relations* 46, (no. 3): 481–510, doi: 10.1111/j.1468-232x.2007.00478.x

6   Mental Health Foundation, 2021, *Stigma and discrimination*, https://www.mentalhealth.org.uk/a-to-z/s/stigma-and-discrimination; Kaushik, A., Kostaki, E., and Kyriakopoulos M., 'The stigma of mental illness in children and adolescents: A systematic review' in *Psychiatry Research* 243 (2016): 469–494, https://doi.org/10.1016/j.psychres.2016.04.042; Corrigan, P., 'How Clinical Diagnosis Might Exacerbate the Stigma of Mental Illness' in *Social Work* 52, no. 1 (2007); 31–39, doi: 10.1093/sw/52.1.31; Mannarini, S., and Rossi, A., 'Assessing Mental Illness Stigma: A Complex Issue' in *Frontiers In Psychology* 9 (2019): doi: 10.3389/fpsyg.2018.02722

Notes

7   Safe Work Australia, 'Mental Health'.

8   Dorter, J., 2019, *The impact of Psychosocial factors on Mental Health and their implications in Life Insurance*; Financial Services Council, https://www.fsc.org.au/news/psychosocial-fsc-kpmg ; TAL, 'Our partners', https://www.tal.com.au/about-us/our-commitments/our-partners, (14 October 2019)

9   Dorter, J., 2019, *The impact of Psychosocial factors on Mental Health and their implications in Life Insurance*; TAL, 'Our partners'; Life Insurance Industry, Life Insurance Industry Response To: Productivity Commission's Draft Report on the Social & Economic Benefits of Improving Mental Health (23 January 2020), https://www.pc.gov.au/__data/assets/pdf_file/0008/250991/sub821-mental-health.pdf

10 Sharma, T., Guski, L.S., Freund, N., et al., 2016, 'Suicidality and aggression during antidepressant treatment: systematic review and meta-analyses based on clinical study reports' in *British Medical Journal (BMJ)* 352: i65: 1–10, https://doi.org/10.1136/bmj.i65; Davies, J., and Read, J., 2019, 'A systematic review into the incidence, severity and duration of antidepressant withdrawal effects: Are guidelines evidence-based?' in *Addictive Behaviors* 97 (2019): 111–121, https://doi.org/10.1016/j.addbeh.2018.08.027

11 Frances, A., 'Why are antidepressants so overprescribed? And what to do about it?', *Health Watch*, published 22 April 2021, https://www.healthwatch-uk.org/publications/newsletter/newsletter-115/231-115-antidepressants.html; Blackburn, P., 'The ERNI Declaration: Making Sense of Distress Without "Disease"', *Mad in America*, published 22 May 2021, https://www.madinamerica.com/2021/05/erni-declaration/?mc_cid=44ac4abae9&mc_eid=babba0de00.

12 Australian Institute of Health and Welfare (AIHW), *Mental health services in Australia: Mental health-related prescriptions*, (Canberra: AIWH, 2019), https://www.aihw.gov.au/reports/mental-health-services/mental-health-services-in-australia/report-contents/mental-health-related-prescriptions

13 Mulder, R., 2008, 'An Epidemic of Depression or the Medicalization of Distress?' in *Perspectives in Biology and Medicine* 51, no. 2: 238–250, doi:10.1353/pbm.0.0009

14 ABS Mental health 2017/18 financial year https://www.abs.gov.au/statistics/health/mental-health/mental-health/latest-release

15 Parker, G., 2007, 'Is depression overdiagnosed? Yes', *BMJ*, doi:10.1136/bmj.39268.475799.AD

16 Australian Government Department of Health, *Summary of consultation with stakeholders – Mental health in Australia* (Canberra: Commonwealth of Australia); The Royal Australian College of General Practitioners, 'DH16 – Doctors' health contextual unit', 2016, https://www.racgp.org.au/education/education-providers/curriculum/contextual-units/populations/dh16-doctors%E2%80%99-health; Australian Medical Association (AMA), 'Health and wellbeing of doctors and medical students – 2020', 14 July 2020, https://www.ama.com.au/position-statement/health-and-wellbeing-doctors-and-medical-students-2020; Cohen, D., and Rhydderch, M., 2006, 'Measuring a doctor's performance: Personality, health and well-being', in *Occupational Medicine* 56, no. 7: 438–40, https://doi.org/10.1093/occmed/kql076; Elliot, L., Tan, J., and Norris, S., 2010, *The mental health of doctors: A systematic literature review*, Hawthorn West, Victoria: Beyond Blue

17 Bagby, R.M., Ryder, A.G., Schuller, D.R., et al., 2004, 'The Hamilton Depression Rating Scale: Has the Gold Standard Become a Lead Weight?' in *American Journal of Psychiatry* 161, no. 12: 2163–2177, doi: 10.1176/appi.ajp.161.12.2163

18 Macintyre, A., Ferris, D., Gonçalves, B. and Quinn, N., 2018, 'What has economics got to do with it? The impact of socioeconomic factors on mental health and the case for collective action' in *Palgrave Communications* 4, no. 1, doi: 10.1057/s41599-018-0063-2; Smith, M., 2016, 'A fine balance: individualism, society and the prevention of mental illness in the United States, 1945–1968' in *Palgrave Communications* 2 https://doi.org/10.1057/palcomms.2016.24; Shim, R., Koplan, C., Langheim, F., et al., 2014, 'The social determinants of mental health: an overview

and call to action' in *Psychiatric Analysis* 44, no. 1 (2014):22–26, https://doi.org/10.3928/00485713-20140108-04

19   Male Suicide Prevention Australia, *The Situational Approach to Suicide Prevention and Mental Health Literacy – Challenging the Deficits of the Current Orthodoxy*, Australian Institute of Male Health and Studies, http://malesuicidepreventionaustralia.com.au/wp-content/uploads/2017/09/Situational-Approach-%E2%80%93-Challenging-the-Deficits.pdf

20   Whitely, M., 2021, *Overprescribing Madness: What's driving Australia's mental illness epidemic?* Melbourne: Wilkinson Publishing

21   Royal Commission into Victoria's Mental Health System, *Final Report, Summary and recommendations*, Melbourne: State of Victoria, February 2021, https://finalreport.rcvmhs.vic.gov.au/download-report/; Timimi, S., 'Mainstream mental health services are a disaster', accessed 30 Nov 2022http://www.uncancelled.co.uk/health/mainstream-mental-health-services-are-a-disaster'

22   ABS, '4329.0.00.006 – *Mortality of People Using Mental Health Services and Prescription Medications, Analysis of 2011 data'*, 8 September 2017 https://www.abs.gov.au/ausstats/abs@.nsf/0/EB5F81AAC6462C72CA2581B40012A37D?Opendocument

Chapter 1 – The limits of the current approach to suicide prevention

1   McPhedran, S., and De Leo, D., 2013, 'Miseries suffered, unvoiced, unknown? Communication of suicidal intent by men in "rural" Queensland, Australia' in *Suicide and Life-Threatening Behavior: 5*, https://doi.org/10.1111/sltb.12041; ABS, '4329.0.00.006 – Mortality of People Using Mental Health Services and Prescription Medications, Analysis of 2011 data'

2   Male Suicide Prevention Australia, *The Situational Approach to Suicide Prevention and Mental Health Literacy*

3   World Health Organization (WHO), 2014, 'Preventing suicide: a global imperative' (Geneva: WHO), https://www.who.int/publications/i/item/9789241564779

4   Stone, D.M., Holland, K.M. and Bartholow, B., 2017, *Preventing Suicide: A Technical Package of Policy, Programs, and Practices* (Atlanta, Georgia: National Center for Injury Prevention and Control, Centers for Disease Control and Prevention) https://www.cdc.gov/violenceprevention/pdf/suicidetechnicalpackage.pdf; Public Health Agency of Canada, *Working Together to Prevent Suicide in Canada: the 2016 Progress Report on the Federal Framework for Suicide Prevention* (Government of Canada, December 2016), https://www.canada.ca/en/public-health/services/publications/healthy-living/2016-progress-report-federal-framework-suicide-prevention.html; UK Government Department of Health and Social Care, 'First ever cross-government suicide prevention plan published', *GOV.UK*, 22 January 2019, https://www.gov.uk/government/news/first-ever-cross-government-suicide-prevention-plan-published

5   Suicide Prevention Australia (SPA), 'Suicide prevention gets the attention it deserves during the Federal Budget' (media release, 3 April 2019), https://www.suicidepreventionaust.org/suicide-prevention-gets-the-attention-it-deserves-during-the-federal-budget/

6   Australian Government Department of Health and Ageing, 'Commonwealth response to "The hidden toll: suicide in Australia"' (Canberra, Commonwealth of Australia, 2010), https://www1.health.gov.au/internet/publications/publishing.nsf/Content/mental-pubs-c-toll-toc~mental-pubs-c-toll-str~mental-pubs-c-toll-str-1

7   ABS, *Causes of Death, Australia* (2020); Australian Bureau of Statistics, '3303.0 – Causes of Death, Australia, 2014', 8 March 2016, https://www.abs.gov.au/AUSSTATS/abs@.nsf/DetailsPage/3303.02014?OpenDocument

8   ABS, *Causes of Death, Australia*

9   KPMG and Mental Health Australia, *Investing to Save: The Economic Benefits for Australia of Investment in Mental Health Reform* (May 2018), https://mhaustralia.org/publication/investing-save-kpmg-and-mental-health-australia-report-may-2018;

Kinchin, I., and Doran, C., 2018, 'The Cost of Youth Suicide in Australia' in *International Journal of Environmental Research and Public Health* 15: 1940, https://www.mdpi.com/1660-4601/15/4/672

10   Naghavi, M., 2016, 'Global, regional, and national burden of suicide mortality 1990 to 2016: systematic analysis for the Global Burden of Disease Study 2016' in *BMJ* 364, doi: 10.1136/bmj.l94

11   Murphy, S.L., Xu, J., Kochanek, K.D. et al., 2018, *Mortality in the United States*, 2017 (Hyattsville, Maryland: National Center for Health Statistics), https://www.cdc.gov/nchs/products/databriefs/db328.htm; Jamie Ducharme, 'U.S. Suicide Rates Are the Highest They've Been Since World War II', in *TIME*, 20 June 2019, https://time.com/5609124/us-suicide-rate-increase

12   Office for National Statistics, 'Suicides in the UK: 2018 registrations', 3 September 2019, https://www.ons.gov.uk/peoplepopulationandcommunity/birthsdeathsandmarriages/deaths/bulletins/suicidesintheunitedkingdom/2018registrations

13   Hjelmeland, H., and Knisek, B., 2017, 'Suicide and Mental Disorders: A Discourse of Politics, Power, and Vested Interests' in Death Studies 41: 481–492, https://doi.org/10.1080/07481187.2017.1332905

14   ibid.

15   United Nations. *'Depression: Let's talk about how we address mental health United Nations Human Rights – Office of the High Commissioner'*, 2017, https://www.ohchr.org/EN/NewsEvents/Pages/DisplayNews.aspx?NewsID=21480&LangID=E

16   Whitely, M., 2021, *Overprescribing Madness: What's driving Australia's mental illness epidemic?* Melbourne: Wilkinson Publishing

17   Raven, R., 2012, 'Depression and antidepressants in Australia and beyond – a critical public health analysis', (PhD thesis, University of Wollongong), https://ro.uow.edu.au/theses/3686

18   Department of Health, '2019–20 Federal Budget aldvances long term national health plan'; New South Wales Government Department of Health, 'Record $19.7 million for suicide prevention and expanded mental health services', (media release, 18 June 2019); https://www.health.nsw.gov.au/news/Pages/20190618_04.aspx; health.vic, 'Suicide prevention in Victoria', (Melbourne: State of Victoria), https://www2.health.vic.gov.au/mental-health/prevention-and-promotion/suicide-prevention-in-victoria

19   Beyond Blue, *Annual Highlights 18/19* (Melbourne: 2019), https://www.beyondblue.org.au/docs/default-source/default-document-library/beyond-blue-annual-highlights-2018-19-web.pdf; Black Dog Institute, Annual Report 2018–2019 (Randwick, NSW: 2019), https://www.blackdoginstitute.org.au/docs/default-source/annual-reports/black-dog-annual-report-2018-19.pdf?sfvrsn=0

20   Australian Government Department of Health, 'Additional $20 million for Mental Health and Suicide Prevention Research 2020' (media release, 25 May 2020), https://www.health.gov.au/ministers/the-hon-greg-hunt-mp/media/additional-20-million-for-mental-health-and-suicide-prevention-research; Australian Government Department of Health, 'Million Minds Mental Health Research Mission', accessed 10 February 2021, https://www.health.gov.au/initiatives-and-programs/million-minds-mental-health-research-mission

21   Lilienfeld, S.O., 2015, 'Introduction to Special Section on Pseudoscience in Psychiatry' in *Canadian Journal of Psychiatry* 60, no, 12: 531–533, https://journals.sagepub.com/doi/10.1177/070674371506001202 ; Ross, C.A., and Alvin, P., 1995, *Pseudoscience in biological psychiatry*, New York: John Wiley & Son

22   Pūras, D., 2017, *Report of the Special Rapporteur on the right of everyone to the enjoyment of the highest attainable standard of physical and mental health*, United Nations Human Rights Council Thirty-fifth session, https://reliefweb.int/report/world/report-special-rapporteur-right-everyone-enjoyment-highest-attainable-standard-0

23 White J. and Morris J., 2019, 'Re-Thinking Ethics and Politics in Suicide Prevention: Bringing Narrative Ideas into Dialogue with Critical Suicide Studies' in *Int. J Environ Res Public Health*. 4;16(18):3236

24 Special Rapporteur, '*Open Statement by the Special Rapporteur on the right of everyone to the enjoyment of the highest attainable standard of physical and mental health*', United Nations Human Rights: Office of the High Commissioner, 10 October 2019, https://www.ohchr.org/EN/NewsEvents/Pages/DisplayNews. aspx?NewsID=25117&LangID=E

25 Lebowitz, M., and Appelbaum, P., 2019, 'Biomedical Explanations of Psychopathology and Their Implications for Attitudes and Beliefs About Mental Disorders' in *Annual Review of Clinical Psychology*, 15(1), 555–577. doi: 10.1146/annurev-clinpsy-050718-095416 https://www.ncbi.nlm.nih.gov/pmc/articles/PMC6506347/

26 Whitely, M., 2021, *Overprescribing Madness: What's driving Australia's mental illness epidemic?*, Wilkinson Publishing

27 WHO, 'What are the social determinants of health', accessed 22 June 2020, https://www.who.int/social_determinants/en

28 WHO and Calouste Gulbenkian Foundation, *Integrating the response to mental disorders and other chronic diseases in health care systems*, Geneva: WHO, 2014, https://apps.who.int/iris/handle/10665/112830.https://www.who.int/mental_health/publications/gulbenkian_paper_social_determinants_of_mental_health/en ; Silva, M., Loureiro, A., and Cardoso, G., 'Social determinants of mental health: A review of the evidence' in European Journal of Psychiatry 30, no. 4 (2016): 259–292, https://psycnet.apa.org/record/2017-05809-003; Shim et al., 'The social determinants of mental health'

29 Friedli, L., Mental health, resilience and inequalities, Copenhagen: WHO Regional Office for Europe, 2009, https://apps.who.int/iris/bitstream/handle/10665/107925/E92227.pdf

30 Australian Government Department of Veteran's Affairs, National Mental Health Commission Review, *Review into the Suicide and Self-Harm Prevention services available to current and former serving ADF members and their families*, Canberra: Commonwealth of Australia, 28 March 2017, 38–39, https://www.dva.gov.au/sites/default/files/files/publications/health/Literature_Review.pdf

31 Knox, K.L., Conwell, Y., and Caine, E.D., 2004, 'If suicide is a public health problem, what are we doing to prevent it?' in *American Journal of Public Health* 94, no. 1: 37–45, doi:10.2105/ajph.94.1.37; Macdonald, J., Smith A., Gethin, A. et al., 'Pathways to despair: a study of male suicide (aged 25–44)', in *Public Health Research* 4, no. 2 (2016): 62–70, https://doi.org/doi:10.5923/j.phr.20140402.03

32 Oliffe, J., and Moodie, R., 'Untangling Men's Depression and Suicide', *The University of Melbourne*, https://pursuit.unimelb.edu.au/articles/untangling-men-s-depression-and-suicide; Australian Institute of Family Studies, 'Depression, suicidality and loneliness: mental health and Australian men' (media release, 16 September 2020), https://aifs.gov.au/media-releases/depression-suicidality-and-loneliness-mental-health-and-australian-men; Trivedi, M., 'Breakthroughs in depression research lead to more effective treatments', UT Southwestern Medical Centre, 9 December 2020, https://utswmed.org/medblog/antidepressants-research-treatments/

33 Shim et al., 'The social determinants of mental health'

34 ABS, '3303.0 – Causes of Death, Australia, 2017', 26 September 2018, https://www.abs.gov.au/ausstats/abs@.nsf/Lookup/by%20Subject/3303.0~2017~Main%20Features~Intentional%20self-harm,%20key%20characteristics~3; Guntuku, S., Hall, N., and Smith, A., 2021, 'Situational Approach to Suicide Prevention Among Australian Males: The Role of Unemployment' in *International Journal Of Social Science Research* 9, no. 1: 93–101, doi: 10.5296/ijssr.v9i1.18168; Haw, C., Hawton, K., Gunnell, D., et al., 2015, 'Economic recession and suicidal behaviour: Possible mechanisms and ameliorating factors', *International Journal of Social Psychiatry* 61, no. 1: 73–81, doi:10.1177/0020764014536545; Nordt, C., Warnke, I., Seifritz, E., et al.,

'Modeling suicide and unemployment: a longitudinal analysis covering 63 countries, 2000–11' in *Lancet Psychiatry* 2, no. 3 (2015): 239–45, https://doi.org/10.1016/S2215-0366(14)00118-7; McPhedran and De Leo, 'Miseries suffered, unvoiced, unknown? Communication of suicidal intent by men in "rural" Queensland, Australia'; see 'Table 1: Intentional Self-Harm Fatalities in Australia by Employment Status and Age Range' in Eva Saar and Thomas Burgess, 'Intentional Self-Harm Fatalities in Australia 2001–2013. Data Report DR16–16 (2016) National Coronial Information System', http://malesuicidepreventionaustralia.com.au/wp-content/uploads/2017/01/NCIS-Report-2016_FINAL.pdf

35   Saar, E., and Burgess, T., 2016, 'Intentional Self-Harm Fatalities in Australia 2001–2013'; Reeves, A., et al., 'Economic shocks, resilience, and male suicides in the Great Recession: cross-national analysis of 20 EU countries', *European Journal of Public Health* 25, no. 3 (2015):404–409, doi: 10.1093/eurpub/cku168

36   Nordt, C. et al., 2015, 'Modelling suicide and unemployment: A longitudinal analysis covering 63 countries, 2000–11,' in *Lancet Psychiatry*, 2(3), pp. 239–245. Available at: https://doi.org/10.1016/s2215-0366(14)00118-7; Haw, C. et al., 2014, 'Economic recession and suicidal behaviour: Possible mechanisms and ameliorating factors', in *International Journal of Social Psychiatry*, 61(1), pp. 73–81. Available at: https://doi.org/10.1177/0020764014536545

37   Fitzpatrick, S.J., 2017, 'Reshaping the Ethics of Suicide Prevention: Responsibility, Inequality and Action on the Social Determinants of Suicide' in *Public Health Ethics* 11, no, 2): 179–190, doi: 10.1093/phe/phx022

38   Ashfield, J., Macdonald, J. and Smith, A., 2017, 'A 'Situational Approach' to Suicide Prevention: Why we need a paradigm shift for effective suicide prevention'. Australian Institute of Male Health and Studies, https://doi.org/10.25155/2017/150417

39   Scott, A., and Guo, B., 2008, 'For which strategies of suicide prevention is there evidence of effectiveness?' Copenhagen, Denmark: WHO Regional Office for Europe http://www.euro.who.int/__data/assets/pdf_file/0005/169466/E96630.pdf

40   Macintyre, A., Ferris, D., Gonçalves, et al., 2018, 'What has economics got to do with it? The impact of socioeconomic factors on mental health and the case for collective action' in *Palgrave Communications*, 4(1). doi: 10.1057/s41599-018-0063-2 https://www.nature.com/articles/s41599-018-0063-2

41   White, J., and Morris, J., 2019, 'Re-Thinking Ethics and Politics in Suicide Prevention: Bringing Narrative Ideas into Dialogue with Critical Suicide Studies' in *International Journal of Environmental Research and Public Health* 16, no. 18 (2019): 3236, https://doi.org/10.3390/ijerph16183236

42   White, J., Marsh, I., Kral, M.J., et al., (eds), 2016, *Critical Suicidology: Transforming Suicide Research and Prevention for the 21st Century*, Vancouver, Canada: UBC Press; Knox, K., 2014, 'Approaching Suicide as a Public Health Issue' in *Annals of Internal Medicine* 161, no. 2: 151–152, doi:10.7326/M14- 0914; Heidi Hjelmeland et al., 'Psychological Autopsy Studies as Diagnostic Tools: Are They Methodologically Flawed?' in *Death Studies* 36, no. 7 (2012): 605–626, doi: 10.1080/07481187.2011.584015; Ross and Pam, *Pseudoscience in biological psychiatry*; Lilienfeld, 'Introduction to Special Section on Pseudoscience in Psychiatry'

43   Fitzpatrick, S J., 'Reshaping the Ethics of Suicide Prevention'; Knox, K., 'Approaching Suicide as a Public Health Issue'

44   ABS, '3303.0–Causes of Death, Australia, 2017'

45   Hjelmeland, H., Dieserud, G., Dyregrov, et al., 2012, 'Psychological Autopsy Studies as Diagnostic Tools: Are they methodologically flawed?' in Death Studies, 36(7), pp. 605–626. Available at: https://doi.org/10.1080/07481187.2011.584015

46   Public Health Information Development Unit (PHIDU), 'Social Health Atlases: Social Health Atlases of Australia: Local Government Areas', Adelaide: Torrens University Australia, accessed 10 December 2019, http://phidu.torrens.edu.au/social-health-atlases/maps#social-health-atlases-of-australia-local-government-areas

47   ABS, 'Causes of Death, Australia, 2018', 25 September 2019, https://www.abs.gov.au/
       statistics/health/causes-death/causes-death-australia/2018

48   Canetto, S. and Sakinofsky, I., 1998, 'The gender paradox in suicide' in *Suicide and
       Life-Threatening Behavior,* 28, no. 1:1; Australian Institute of Health and Welfare,
       Suicide and intentional self-harm, Canberra: AIHW, 23 July 2020, https://www.aihw.
       gov.au/reports/australias-health/suicide-and-intentional-self-harm

49   Harrison, J., and Henley, G., *Suicide and hospitalised self-harm in Australia: trends
       and analysis,* Canberra: AIHW; 2014, 58, https://www.aihw.gov.au/reports/
       australias-health/suicide-and-intentional-self-harm

50   Hawton, K., Zahl, D., and Weatherall R., 2003, 'Suicide following deliberate self-
       harm: long-term follow-up of patients who presented to a general hospital', in *British
       Journal of Psychiatry* 182:537–542

51   Owens, D., Horrocks. J., and House, A., 2002, 'Fatal and non-fatal repetition of self-
       harm. Systematic review' in *British Journal of Psychiatry*;181:193–199

52   Isometsa, E.T., and Lonnqvist J.K., 1998, 'Suicide attempts preceding completed
       suicide' in *British Journal of Psychiatry*:173:531-5, 531 (Conclusions: Most male and a
       substantial proportion of female suicides die in their first suicide attempt.)

53   McPhedran, S., and De Leo, D., 2013, 'Miseries suffered, unvoiced, unknown?
       Communication of suicidal intent by men in "rural" Queensland, Australia', *Suicide
       and Life-Threatening Behavior,* 43(6), 589–597. Available at: https://doi.org/10.1111/
       sltb.12041

54   Hjelmeland, H., et al., 'Psychological Autopsy Studies as Diagnostic Tools'

55   Bertolote, J.M. and Fleischmann, A., 2002, 'Suicide and psychiatric diagnosis: a
       worldwide perspective', *World psychiatry* 1, no.3:181–185

56   Grundy, Q., et al., 2017, *Finding Peace of Mind: Navigating the Marketplace of Mental
       Health Apps,* Sydney: Australian Communications Consumer Action Network;
       Leigh, S. and Flatt, S., 2015, 'App-based psychological interventions: friend or foe?'
       in *BMJ Evidence-Based Mental Health* 18, no. 4: 97–99, doi: 10.1136/eb-2015-102203;
       Lisa Parker et al., 'Mental Health Messages in Prominent Mental Health Apps' in
       Annals of Family Medicine 16, no. 4 (2018): 338–342, doi: 10.1370/afm.2260; Jutel, A.,
       and Lupton, D., 2015, 'Digitizing diagnosis: a review of mobile applications in the
       diagnostic process' in *Diagnosis* 2, no. 2: 89–96, doi: 10.1515/dx-2014-0068; Larsen,
       M.E. et al., 2019, 'Using science to sell apps: Evaluation of mental health app store
       quality claims' in *npj Digital Medicine* 2, no.18, doi:10.1038/s41746-019-0093-1

57   Lagan, S., D'Mello, R., Vaidyam, A., et al., 2021, 'Assessing mental health apps
       marketplaces with objective metrics from 29,190 data points from 278 apps' in
       Acta Psychiatrica Scandinavica, 144(2), pp. 201–210. Available at: https://doi.
       org/10.1111/acps.13306. Friedman, E., 'The Mental Health App Marketplace is a
       Mess, Researchers Find', *Mad in America,* 24 April 2021, https://www.madinamerica.
       com/2021/04/mental-health-app-marketplace-mess-researchers-find/

58   Demasi, M., and Gøtzsche, P., 2020, 'Presentation of benefits and harms of
       antidepressants on websites: A cross-sectional study' in *International Journal of Risk
       & Safety In Medicine,* 31(2), 53-65. doi: 10.3233/jrs-19102

Chapter 2 – Distress as clinical disorder:
a history and critique of the clinical approach to depression and anxiety

1   AIHW, 2019, *Mental health services—in brief 2019. Cat. no. HSE 228,* Canberra: AIHW,
       https://www.aihw.gov.au/getmedia/f7395726-55e6-4e0a-9c1c-01f3ab67c193/aihw-
       hse-228-in-brief.pdf.aspx?inline=true

2   Horwitz, A., 2010, 'How an age of anxiety became an age of depression', *Milbank
       Quarterly* 88, no. 1: 112–138, doi:10.1111/j.1468-0009.2010.00591.x; Healy, D., 2006,
       Let Them Eat Prozac, NYU Press; Healy, D., 2004, 'Shaping the Intimate: Influence on
       the Experience of Everyday Nerves' in *Social Studies of Science* 34, no. 2: 219–245;

Notes

Harrington, A., 2019, *Mind Fixers: Psychiatry's Troubled Search for the Biology of Mental Illness*, New York: W.W. Norton & Company; Selye, H., 1968, *The Stress of Life*, New York, McGraw Hill; Herzberg, D., 2009, *Happy Pills in America: From Miltown to Prozac*, Baltimore: Johns Hopkins University Press; Olfson, M., et al., 2002, 'National Trends in the Outpatient Treatment of Depression' in *Journal of the American Medical Association* 287: 203–9; Kolb, L., Frazier, S.H., and Sirovatka, P., 2000, 'The National Institute of Mental Health: Its Influence on Psychiatry and the Nation's Mental Health', in *American Psychiatry after World War II: 1944–1994*, eds. R.W. Menninger and J.C. Nemiah, Washington, DC: American Psychiatric Press, 207–231

3   ABS, *National Survey of Mental Health and Wellbeing: Summary of Results*, Belconnen, ACT: Commonwealth of Australia, 23 October 2008, https://www.abs.gov.au/statistics/health/mental-health/national-survey-mental-health-and-wellbeing-summary-results/latest-release

4   Center for Epidemiologic Studies, 'Depression Scale (CES-D), NIMH', https://www.apa.org/depression-guideline/epidemiologic-studies-scale.pdf; 'Hamilton Depression Rating Scale (HAM-D)', adapted from Max Hamilton, *Journal of Neurology, Neurosurgery, and Psychiatry* 23 (1960):56–62, https://www.apa.org/depression-guideline/hamilton-rating-scale.pdf; Douglas, M., Maurer, D.M., Tyler, J. et al., 'Depression: Screening and Diagnosis' in *American Family Physician* 98, no. 8 (2018): 508–515, https://www.apa.org/depression-guideline/hamilton-rating-scale.pdf

5   Fried, E., and Nesse, R., 2015, 'Depression sum-scores don't add up: why analyzing specific depression symptoms is essential', in *BMC Medicine* 13, no. 72, doi: 10.1186/s12916-015-0325-4

6   Allsopp, K., Read, J., Corcoran, et al., 2019, 'Heterogeneity in psychiatric diagnostic classification.' In *Psychiatry Research*; 279: 15 DOI: 10.1016/j.psychres.2019.07.005

7   University of Liverpool, 'Psychiatric diagnosis "scientifically meaningless"', ScienceDaily., 8 July 2019, www.sciencedaily.com/releases/2019/07/190708131152.htm

8   Paykel, E., 2008, 'Basic concepts of depression' in *Dialogues in clinical neuroscience* 10, no. 3: 281, https://www.researchgate.net/publication/23447361_Basic_concepts_of_depression

9   Paris, J., 2014, 'The mistreatment of major depressive disorder' in *Canadian Journal of Psychiatry* 59, no. 3: 148–151, doi:10.1177/070674371405900306

10 Pilgrim, D., and Bentall, R., 1999, 'The medicalisation of misery: A critical realist analysis of the concept of depression' in *Journal of Mental Health* 8, no. 3: 261–274, doi: 10.1080/09638239917427

11 Hasler, G., 2010, 'Pathophysiology of depression: do we have any solid evidence of interest to clinicians?' in *World psychiatry* 9, no. 3: 155–161, doi: 10.1002/j.2051-5545.2010.tb00298.x

12 Newson, J., Hunter, D., and Thiagarajan, T., 2020, 'The Heterogeneity of Mental Health Assessment' in *Frontiers In Psychiatry*, 11. doi: 10.3389/fpsyt.2020.00076 https://doi.org/10.3389/fpsyt.2020.00076

13 Moncrieff, M., and Timimi, S., 2013, 'The social and cultural construction of psychiatric knowledge: an analysis of NICE guidelines on depression and ADHD' in *Anthropology & Medicine* 20, no. 1: 59–71, DOI: 10.1080/13648470.2012.747591

14 MacQueen, G., Santaguida, P., and Keshavarz, H., et al., 2017, 'Systematic Review of Clinical Practice Guidelines for Failed Antidepressant Treatment Response in Major Depressive Disorder, Dysthymia, and Subthreshold Depression in Adults' in *Canadian Journal of Psychiatry* 62, no. 1:11–23, doi:10.1177/0706743716664885

15 Zafra-Tanaka, J.H., Goicochea-Lugo, S., and Villarreal-Zegarra, D., et al., 2019, 'Characteristics and quality of clinical practice guidelines for depression in adults: a scoping review' *BMC Psychiatry* 19, no. 1, doi:10.1186/s12888-019-2057-z

169

16   Kirk, S., and Kutchins, H., 1994 'The myth of reliability of DSM' in *Journal of Mind and Behavior* 15: 71–86, https://www.researchgate.net/publication/232558296_The_myth_of_reliability_of_DSM

17   Dowrick, C., and Frances, A., 2013, 'Medicalising unhappiness: new classification of depression risks more patients being put on drug treatment from which they will not benefit' in *BMJ* 347, no. f7140, doi: 10.1136/bmj.f7140

18   Keshavarz, H., Fitzpatrick-Lewis, D., Streiner, et al., 2013, 'Screening for depression: a systematic review and meta-analysis' in *CMAJ Open* 1, no. 4, doi:10.9778/cmajo.20130030

19   Roseman, M., Kloda, LA., Saadat, N., et al., 2016, 'Accuracy of Depression Screening Tools to Detect Major Depression in Children and Adolescents: A Systematic Review', *The Canadian Journal of Psychiatry* 61, no. 12: 746–757, doi: 10.1177/0706743716651833

20   Cosgrove, L., Karter, JM., Vaswani, A. et al., 2018, 'Unexamined assumptions and unintended consequences of routine screening for depression' in *Journal of Psychosomatic Research* 109: 9–11, DOI: 10.1016/j.jpsychores.2018.03.007

21   Hopwood, M., and Malhi, G., 2016, 'To screen for depression or not?' in *The Medical Journal of Australia* 204, no. 9, doi: 10.5694/mja16.00217

22   Pilgrim, D., and Bentall, R., 1999, 'The medicalisation of misery: A critical realist analysis of the concept of depression' in *Journal of Mental Health* 8, no. 3: 261–274, doi: 10.1080/09638239917427

23   Deacon, B., 2013, 'The biomedical model of mental disorder: A critical analysis of its validity, utility, and effects on psychotherapy research' in *Clinical Psychology Review* 33, no. 7: 846–861, doi: 10.1016/j.cpr.2012.09.007

24   ibid.

25   Burton, N., 'Criticisms of the Concept of Depression', published 25 March 2011, https://neelburton.com/2011/03/25/criticisms-of-the-concept-of-depression

26   Hanson, N., Owens, M. J. and Nemeroff, C. B., 2011, 'Depression, Antidepressants, and Neurogenesis: A Critical Reappraisal' in *Neuropsychopharmacology* 36, no. 13: 2589–2602, doi: 10.1038/npp.2011.220

27   Hopwood and Malhi, 'To screen for depression or not?' 129

28   Mulder, 'An Epidemic of Depression or the Medicalization of Distress?'

29   Horwitz, A., 2010, 'How an age of anxiety became an age of depression', *Milbank Quarterly*, 88(1), pp. 112–138. Available at: https://doi.org/10.1111/j.1468-0009.2010.00591.x. Healy, D., 2003, *Let Them Eat Prozac*, Toronto: J. Lorimer & Co.; Healy, D., 'Shaping the Intimate'; Harrington, *Mind Fixers*; Selye, *The Stress of Life*; Herzberg, *Happy Pills in America*; Olfson, et al., 'National Trends in the Outpatient Treatment of Depression'; Kolb, Frazier and Sirovatka, 'The National Institute of Mental Health'

30   Paykel, 'Basic concepts of depression', 281

31   Horwitz, 'How an age of anxiety became an age of depression'; Shorter, E., *Before Prozac: The Troubled History of Mood Disorders in Psychiatry.*(New York: Oxford University Press, 2008

32   Horwitz, 'How an age of anxiety became an age of depression'

33   ibid., 113

34   ibid.

35   ibid.

36   Hengartner, M., and Plöderl, M., 2018, 'Statistically significant antidepressant-placebo differences on subjective symptom-rating scales do not prove that the drugs work: Effect size and method bias matter!' in *Frontiers in Psychiatry* 9. doi: 10.3389/fpsyt.2018.00517

37   Moncrieff, J., 2007, 'Are Antidepressants as Effective as Claimed? No, They are Not Effective at All' in *Canadian Journal Of Psychiatry* 52, no. 2: 96–97, doi: 10.1177/070674370705200204

38   Turner, E.H., Matthews, A.M., Linardatos, E., et al., 2008, 'Selective Publication of Antidepressant Trials and Its Influence on Apparent Efficacy' in New England Journal of Medicine 358, no. 3: 252–260, doi: 10.1056/nejmsa065779

39   Hengartner, M., 2017, 'Methodological flaws, conflicts of interest, and scientific fallacies: Implications for the evaluation of antidepressants' efficacy and harm' in *Frontiers of Psychiatry* 8, doi: 10.3389/fpsyt.2017.00275

40   Horwitz, 'How an age of anxiety became an age of depression'

41   Paykel, 'Basic concepts of depression', 280

42   Horwitz, 'How an age of anxiety became an age of depression'

43   Frances, A., 2013, 'Saving normal: An insider's revolt against out-of-control psychiatric diagnosis, DSM-5, big pharma and the medicalization of ordinary life', *Psychotherapy in Australia* 19, no. 3: 14–18

44   Rief, W., and Martin, A., 2014, 'How to Use the New DSM-5 Somatic Symptom Disorder Diagnosis in Research and Practice: A Critical Evaluation and a Proposal for Modifications' in *Annual Review of Clinical Psychology* 10, no 1: 339–367, doi: 10.1146/annurev-clinpsy-032813-153745

45   Tyrer, P., 2014, 'A comparison of DSM and ICD classifications of mental disorder' in *Advances in Psychiatric Treatment* 20, no. 4: 280–285, doi: 10.1192/apt.bp.113.011296

46   Fried, E., 2017, 'The 52 symptoms of major depression: lack of content overlap among seven common depression scales' in *Journal of Affective Disorders* 208, doi: 10.1016/j.jad.2016.10.019; Fried and Nesse, 'Depression sum-scores don't add up'; Hasler, 'Pathophysiology of depression'; Paykel, 'Basic concepts of depression'

47   Timimi, S., 2013, 'No More Psychiatric Labels: Campaign to Abolish Psychiatric Diagnostic Systems such as ICD and DSM (CAPSID)', *Self & Society* 40, no. 4: 6–14, doi: 10.1080/03060497.2013.11084297

48   Lebowitz, M., and Appelbaum, P., 2019, 'Biomedical Explanations of Psychopathology and Their Implications for Attitudes and Beliefs About Mental Disorders', in *Annual Review of Clinical Psychology* 15, no. 1: 555–577, doi: 10.1146/annurev-clinpsy-050718-095416

49   Newson, J.J., Hunter, D. and Thiagarajan, T. C., 2020, 'The Heterogeneity of Mental Health Assessment' in *Frontiers of Psychiatry* 11, doi: 10.3389/fpsyt.2020.00076

50   WHO, *Depression and Other Common Mental Disorders: Global Health Estimates*, Geneva: WHO, 2017, https://apps.who.int/iris/bitstream/handle/10665/254610/WHO-MSD-MER-2017.2-eng.pdf

51   ibid., 8

52   ibid., 10

53   Blue Cross Blue Shield Association, 'Major Depression: The Impact on Overall Health', 10 May 2018, https://www.bcbs.com/the-health-of-america/reports/major-depression-the-impact-overall-health

54   UK Council for Psychotherapy, 'Depression and anxiety up by almost a third among workers', (media release, accessed 20 August 2020); Mental Health Foundation, *Fundamental Facts About Mental Health 2016* (London: 2016), 14, https://www.mentalhealth.org.uk/sites/default/files/fundamental-facts-about-mental-health-2016.pdf; Evans, J., Macrory, I. and Randall, C., 2016, 'Measuring national well-being: Life in the UK, 2016' (Office for National Statistics, 23 March 2016), ons.gov.uk/peoplepopulationandcommunity/wellbeing/articles/measuringnationalwellbeing/2016#how-good-is-our-health

55   Wilkins, R., Lass, I., Butterworth, P. et al., 2019, 'Living in Australia: A snapshot of Australian society and how it is changing over time', *Melbourne Institute: Applied Economic & Social Research, University of Melbourne*, 27–29, https://

melbourneinstitute.unimelb.edu.au/__data/assets/pdf_file/0005/3126038/
LivingInAus-2019.pdf

56 Wilkins et al., 'The Household, Income and Labour Dynamics in Australia Survey'
57 Lawrence D., Johnson, S., Hafekost J., et al., 2015, *The Mental Health of Children and
    Adolescents. Report on the second Australian Child and Adolescent Survey of Mental
    Health and Wellbeing.* Department of Health, Canberra, http://www.health.gov.au/
    internet/main/publishing.nsf/content/9DA8CA21306FE6EDCA257E2700016945/$
    File/child2.pdf
58 The Royal Australian and New Zealand Collage of Psychiatrists (RANZP), *The
    economic cost of serious mental illness and comorbidities in Australia and New Zealand*
    (2016), https://www.ranzcp.org/files/resources/reports/ranzcp-serious-mental-
    illness.aspx
59 ibid., 15
60 'Workplace mental health claims on the rise', in *Mirage*, 2 September 2020,
    https://www.miragenews.com/workplace-mental-health-claims-on-the-rise;
    Grieve, C., '"Looming crisis": Insurers brace for surge in mental health claims',
    in *Sydney Morning Herald*, 27 July 2020, https://www.smh.com.au/business/
    banking-and-finance/looming-crisis-insurers-brace-for-surge-in-mental-health-
    claims-20200727-p55ftn.html
61 Mental Health Foundation, 'Stigma and discrimination'
62 Kaushik, A., Kostaki, E. and Kyriakopoulos, M., 2016, 'The stigma of mental illness
    in children and adolescents: A systematic review' in *Psychiatry Research*, 243, pp.
    469–494. Available at: https://doi.org/10.1016/j.psychres.2016.04.042
63 Corrigan', P.W., 2007, 'How clinical diagnosis might exacerbate the stigma of mental
    illness', in *Social Work*, 52(1), pp. 31–39. Available at: https://doi.org/10.1093/
    sw/52.1.31; Mannarini, S., and Rossi, A., 2019, 'Assessing Mental Illness Stigma: A
    Complex Issue' in *Front Psychol.* 11;9:2722. doi: 10.3389/fpsyg.2018.02722. PMID:
    30687177; PMCID: PMC6336735.
64 Fox, A., et al., 2018, 'Conceptualizing and measuring mental illness stigma: The
    mental illness stigma framework and critical review of measures' in *Stigma and
    Health* 3, no. 4: 348–376, doi: 10.1037/sah0000104
65 Bezborodovs, N. and Thornicroft, G., 2013, 'Stigmatisation of mental illness in the
    workplace: evidence and consequences' in *Die Psychiatrie* 10, no. 2: 102–107, doi:
    10.1055/s-0038-1670862
66 Benenden Health, 'The elephant that never left the room: Why
    stigma is still preventing employees from telling their boss the truth
    about their mental wellbeing in the workplace', York: The Benenden
    Healthcare Society Limited, September 2020, https://www.benenden.
    co.uk/media/6907/benenden-mental-wellbeing-report-2020_single.
    pdf?b2b_number=0808+252+0628&campaign_code=SALES&benenden_campaign=1
67 Keenan, C., 'How Insurers Discriminate Against People With Mental
    Health Conditions' in *Junkee*, 15 February 2021, https://junkee.com/
    insurance-industry-found-to-discriminate-against-mental-ill-health/287912
68 Link, B.G., Wells, J., Phelan, J.C. et al., 2015, 'Understanding the Importance of
    "Symbolic Interaction Stigma": How Expectations About the Reactions of Others
    Adds to the Burden of Mental Illness Stigma', in *Psychiatric Rehabilitation Journal* 38,
    no. 2: 117–24, DOI: 10.1037/prj0000142
69 Kenny, A., Bizumic, B., and Griffiths, K.M., 2018, 'The Prejudice towards People with
    Mental Illness (PPMI) scale: structure and validity', in *BMC Psychiatry* 18, no. 293,
    https://doi.org/10.1186/s12888-018-1871-z
70 Horwitz, 'How an age of anxiety became an age of depression'
71 ibid.
72 Horwitz, 'How an age of anxiety became an age of depression'; Herzberg, *Happy Pills
    in America*

73   ibid.
74   Horwitz, 'How an age of anxiety became an age of depression'; Herzberg, *Happy Pills in America*; Olfson, et al., 'National Trends in the Outpatient Treatment of Depression'; IMS America, *National Disease and Therapeutic Index* (Ambler, Pennsylvania: IMS America, 1976)
75   Horwitz, 'How an age of anxiety became an age of depression', 116; Mojtabai, R., 2008, 'Increase in Antidepressant Medication in the US Adult Population between 1990 and 2003', in *Psychotherapy and Psychosomatics* 77, no. 2: 83–92, doi: 10.1159/000112885
76   Horwitz, 'How an age of anxiety became an age of depression'; IMS America, *National Disease and Therapeutic Index*
77   Horwitz, 'How an age of anxiety became an age of depression'
78   Deacon, 'The biomedical model of mental disorder'
79   Horwitz, 'How an age of anxiety became an age of depression'; Kolb, Frazier and Sirovatka, 'The National Institute of Mental Health'
80   ibid.
81   Smith, M., 1985, *A Social History of the Minor Tranquillizers*, New York: Pharmaceutical Products Press; Horwitz, 'How an age of anxiety became an age of depression'
82   Azoth Analytics, 2018, *Global Antidepressant Drugs Market – Analysis By Drugs Class, By Sales Channel, By Region, By Country: Opportunities and Forecasts (2018–2023)*
83   BrandEssence Market Research, 'Antidepressant Drugs Market Size, Share, Current trends, Opportunities, Competitive Analysis and Forecast to 2019–2025' (2019)
84   OECD, 'OECD Health Statistics 2018', 28 June 2018, https://www.oecd.org/els/health-systems/health-data.htm; Michael McCarthy, 'Antidepressant use has doubled in rich nations in past 10 years', in *BMJ* 347, no. f7261 (2013), doi: https://doi.org/10.1136/bmj.f7261; Australian Government Department of Health: Therapeutic Goods Administration, 'Provisional application receives approval through the first international collaborative review initiative between TGA, FDA and HC', (media release, 25 September 2019), https://www.tga.gov.au/media-release/provisional-application-receives-approval-through-first-international-collaborative-review-initiative-between-tga-fda-and-hc
85   Anxiety and Depression Association of America, 'Facts & Statistics', accessed 21 August 2020, https://adaa.org/about-adaa/press-room/facts-statistics; National Institute of Mental Health, 'Statistics', accessed 7 August 2019, https://www.nimh.nih.gov/health/statistics/index.shtml
86   Beyond Blue, 'Anxiety', https://www.beyondblue.org.au/the-facts/anxiety
87   Tyrer, P., 2018, 'Against the Stream: Generalised anxiety disorder (GAD) – a redundant diagnosis', in *BJPsych Bulletin* 42, no. 2: 69–71, doi: 10.1192/bjb.2017.12
88   Tyrer, 'Against the Stream: Generalised anxiety disorder (GAD) – a redundant diagnosis'
89   ibid.
90   Tyrer, 'Against the Stream: Generalised anxiety disorder (GAD) – a redundant diagnosis'; ABS, National Survey of Mental Health and Wellbeing: Summary of Results, 67–68;70; Anxiety Disorder Association of America, *Generalised Anxiety Disorder* (2015) https://adaa.org/sites/default/files/July%2015%20GAD_adaa.pdf
91   Harrington, *Mind Fixers*
92   National Institute of Mental Health, 'Statistics'
93   AIHW, *Mental health services in Australia: Mental health-related prescriptions*

Chapter 3 – The role of the mental health sector

1   'The Shed', Western Sydney University, https://www.westernsydney.edu.au/mhirc/mens_health_information_and_resource_centre/our_work/research_projects/the_shed

2   Robinson, J. and Cox, G.R., 'Can barriers prevent suicide or do they just shift the problem?', In *Conversation*, 1 March 2012, https://theconversation.com/can-barriers-prevent-suicide-or-do-they-just-shift-the-problem-5515

3   Raven, 'Depression and antidepressants in Australia and Beyond', 339

4   Whitely, M., Raven, M. and Jureidini, J., 2020, 'Antidepressant prescribing and suicide/self-harm by Young Australians: Regulatory warnings, contradictory advice, and long-term trends', in *Frontiers in Psychiatry*, 11. Available at https://doi.org/10.3389/fpsyt.2020.00478

5   Whitely, *Overprescribing Madness*

6   Raven, 'Depression and antidepressants in Australia and Beyond', 379

7   ibid.

8   Royal Commission into Victoria's Mental Health System, *Final Report*

9   Timimi, 'Mainstream mental health services are a disaster'

10 Raven, M., 'Royal Commission into Victoria's Mental Health System submission', http://rcvmhs.archive.royalcommission.vic.gov.au/Raven_Melissa.pdf

11 Jureidini, J., McHenry, L.B., 2020, *The illusion of evidence-based medicine: Exposing the crisis of credibility in Clinical Research*. Adelaide: Wakefield Press; Raven, 'Depression and antidepressants in Australia and Beyond'; Whitely, *Overprescribing Madness*

12 Raven, 'Depression and antidepressants in Australia and Beyond', 302

13 Pirkis, J., Hickie, I., Young. L., et al., 2005, 'An Evaluation of *beyondblue*, Australia's National Depression Initiative' in *International Journal of Health Promotion*, https://doi.org/10.1080/14623730.2005.9721865

14 Beyondblue, Media Release – 'Treatment rates for mental health conditions soar', 2014; cited in Adams, K., Halacas, C., Cincotta, et al., 2014, 'Mental health and Victorian Aboriginal people: what can data mining tell us?' *Australian Journal of Primary Health* 20, 350–355. https://doi.org/10.1071/PY14036

15 Beyond Blue, *Annual Highlights 18/19*, 31; 38

16 Beyond Blue, *Annual Report 2004–2005*, https://www.beyondblue.org.au/about-us/annual-reports; Beyond Blue, '20 years of Beyond Blue', https://www.beyondblue.org.au/about-us/who-we-are-and-what-we-do/20-years-of-beyond-blue

17 Workplace Mental Health Institute, 'Mental Health First Aid Australia: Metal Health First Aid', accessed 7 May 2020, https://www.wmhi.com.au/mental-health-first-aid; Firstaidpro, 'Mental health – Recognising the signs – awareness training', https://www.firstaidpro.com.au/course/MHRSAT

18 Doggett, J., 'The personal and the political: Why do we find it so hard to direct mental health spending to the people who most need it?' in *Inside Story*, 15 June 2019, https://insidestory.org.au/the-personal-and-the-political/

19 Stark, J., and Fyfe., 'What lies beyond?' in *Sydney Morning Herald*, 9 October 2011, https://www.smh.com.au/national/what-lies-beyond-20111008-1lf37.html; Barbour, L., 'Criticism for mental health road show', *ABC Rural*, 28 February 2014, https://www.abc.net.au/news/rural/2014-02-28/criticism-of-beyond-blue-road-show/5290258; Middleton, K., 'Lobbyists dominate mental health sector', in *Saturday Paper*, 6–12 October 2018, https://www.thesaturdaypaper.com.au/news/politics/2018/10/06/lobbyists-dominate-mental-health-sector/15387480006960; 'Casino, depression not in conflict: Kennett', *SBS News*, 3 September 2013, https://www.sbs.com.au/news/casino-depression-not-in-conflict-kennett; Razer, H., 'Razer's Class Warfare: reducing depression's "stigma" is cheap, stupid policy', in *Crikey*, 27 March 2014, http://www.crikey.com.au/2014/03/27/razers-class-warfare-reducing-depressions-stigma-is-cheap-stupid-policy/

Notes

20 Stark and Fyfe, 'What lies beyond?'

21 Australian Government Department of Health and Ageing, 'Commonwealth response to "The hidden toll: suicide in Australia"'

22 Shahtahmasebi, S., 2015, 'Suicide Research: Problems with Interpreting Results' in *Journal of Advances in Medicine and Medical Research* 5, no. 9: 1147–1157, doi: 10.9734/bjmmr/2015/12802

23 Beyond Blue, 'Beyond Blue Chair Julia Gillard delivers 2017 Annual Bob Hawke Lecture', media release, 12 October 2017, https://www.beyondblue.org.au/connect-with-others/news/news/2017/10/12/beyondblue-chair-julia-gillard-delivers-2017-annual-bob-hawke-lecture

24 O'Leary, C., 'WA kids under 7 years old on antidepressants', in *West Australian,* 15 April 2017 https://thewest.com.au/news/wa/wa-kids-under-7-years-old-on-antidepressants-ng-b88445165z; *Today Tonight Adelaide,* 'Kids on Antidepressants – the Alarming Side-effects Parents Aren't Told About', aired 5 May 2017; Beyond Blue, 'Beyond Blue Chair The Hon Julia Gillard, AC, launches Be You' (media release, 1 November 2018), https://www.beyondblue.org.au/media/news/news/2018/10/31/beyond-blue-chair-julia-gillard-launches-be-you.

25 Pūras, *'Report of the Special Rapporteur on the right of everyone to the enjoyment of the highest attainable standard of physical and mental health',* 12

26 Black Dog Institute. 'Workplace Mental Health Toolkit – Practical Guide & Resources' https://www.blackdoginstitute.org.au/wp-content/uploads/2020/04/black-dog-institute-mental-health-toolkit-2017.pdf

27 Ruffalo, M.L., 2014, 'The Medicalization of Suicide' in *Journal of Psychiatry* 17, no. 6, doi: 10.4172/psychiatry.1000e104

28 Ashfield, Macdonald and Smith, A *'Situational Approach'* to Suicide Prevention

29 Whitely, *Overprescribing Madness,* 104

30 Kisely, S. and Looi, J.C.L., 2020, 'Latest evidence casts further doubt on the effectiveness of headspace', in *Medical Journal of Australia,* 217(8), pp. 388–390. Available at: https://doi.org/10.5694/mja2.51700

31 Australian Financial Review, 'Mental health experts question $280m for "abject failure" Headspace', https://www.afr.com/politics/mental-health-experts-question-280m-for-abject-failure-headspace-20210512-p57r7jce

32 Stark, J., and Vedelago, C., 'Headspace: "McDonaldisation" of youth mental healthcare a ticking time bomb' in *Sydney Morning Herald,* 26 April 2015 https://www.smh.com.au/healthcare/headspace-mcdonaldisation-of-youth-mental-healthcare-a-ticking-time-bomb-20150425-1mszey.html

33 Hjelmeland, et al., 'Psychological Autopsy Studies as Diagnostic Tools'

34 ABS, '6362.0 – Employer Training Expenditure and Practices, Australia, 2001–02', 2 April 2003, https://www.abs.gov.au/ausstats/abs@.nsf/mf/6362.0

35 Mental Health First Aid Australia, https://mhfa.com.au

36 Smith, A., 'Focus on individual wellbeing doesn't help', *Guardian,* 8 May 2021, https://www.theguardian.com/society/2021/may/08/the-self-help-cult-of-resilience-teaches-australians-nothing

37 Goff-Deakins, C., 'When resilience training isn't the answer', in *HRZone,* 22 March 2019, https://www.hrzone.com/perform/people/when-resilience-training-isnt-the-answer; Chandrashekar, R., 'The problem with resilience as we know it', in *India Development Review,* 22 October 2020, https://idronline.org/the-problem-with-resilience-as-we-know-it-mental-health-wellbeing/

38 'Resilience', Reachout.com, https://schools.au.reachout.com/resilience?gclid=Cj0KCQjwlouKBhC5ARIsAHXNMI8pu9NT_e6tdz03CjqyRl6SjlZ-rYrOEoqkg4MgS_H53UHRtKI_cJ4aAuYDEALw_wcB

39 Whitely, *Overprescribing Madness,* 174

40   Ashfield, J., and Smith, A., 2018, *The Situational Approach to Suicide Prevention and Mental Health Literacy: Advocating for a new multi-sector and multidisciplinary approach*, 3, http://malesuicidepreventionaustralia.com.au/wp-content/uploads/2018/02/SA-Advocating-for-a-new-multi-sector-approach-190218.pdf

Chapter 4 – Mental health in the workplace: Default Depression in organisational policy and practice

1   WorkSafe WorkWell, 'About WorkWell', accessed 8 May 2020, https://www.workwell.vic.gov.au/about-workwell

2   Beyond Blue, *The beyondblue National Workplace Program: Evaluation results* (2007); Mental Health First Aid Australia, 'Mental Health First Aid'

3   Harvey, S.B., Deady, M., Wang M.J., et al., 2016, 'Is the prevalence of mental illness increasing in Australia? Evidence from national health surveys and administrative data, 2001–2014', in *Medical Journal of Australia* 6, no. 11: 490–493, doi: 10.5694/mja16.00295; Shiels, C. and Gabbay, M.B., 2007, 'Patient, clinician, and general practice factors in long-term certified sickness', in *Scandinavian Journal of Public Health* 35, no. 3 : 250–256, doi: 10.1080/14034940601072364; OECD, 2003, *Transforming Disability into Ability: Policies to Promote Work and Income Security for Disabled People*, Paris: OECD Publishing

4   Gabbay, M., Shiels, C. and Hillage, J., 2016, 'Sickness certification for common mental disorders and GP return-to-work advice', in *Primary Health Care Research & Development*, 17(05), pp. 437–447. Available at: https://doi.org/10.1017/s1463423616000074

5   Harvey, S.B., Deady, M., Wang, M.J., et al., 2016, 'Is the prevalence of mental illness increasing in Australia? Evidence from national health surveys and administrative data, 2001–2014'

6   Dorter, J., 2019, *The impact of Psychosocial factors on Mental Health and their implications in Life Insurance*

7   Life Insurance Industry, *Life Insurance Industry Response To: Productivity Commission's Draft Report on the Social & Economic Benefits of Improving Mental Health*

8   Dorter, J., 2019, *The impact of Psychosocial factors on Mental Health and their implications in Life Insurance*

9   Dembe, A.E., et al., 2003, 'Inpatient hospital care for work-related injuries and illnesses', in *American Journal of Industrial Medicine* 44, no. 4: 331–342, doi:10.1002/ajim.10273

10   ibid., 24

11   Dorter, J., 2019, *The impact of Psychosocial factors on Mental Health and their implications in Life Insurance*

12   Safe Work Australia, 'Mental Health'; Safe Work Australia, *Work-related psychological health and safety: A systematic approach to meeting your duties National Guidance Material* (January 2019), https://www.safeworkaustralia.gov.au/system/files/documents/1911/work-related_psychological_health_and_safety_a_systematic_approach_to_meeting_your_duties.pdf

13   MLC Life Insurance, *'Dealing with depression and anxiety'*

14   Australian Medical Association (AMA), *Mental illness and life insurance: What you need to know – a brief guide*, https://ama.com.au/sites/default/files/documents/Mental_illness_and_life_insurance_a_brief_guide_FINAL2.pdf; headspace, 'How to get a mental health care plan', 13 September 2018, https://headspace.org.au/blog/how-to-get-a-mental-health-care-plan

15   Mazza, et al., *Clinical guideline for the diagnosis and management of work-related mental health conditions in general practice*

16   The Royal Australian College of General Practitioners (RACGP), 'Evidence to guide and support GPs', https://www.racgp.org.au/clinical-resources/clinical-guidelines/

Notes

guidelines-by-topic/endorsed-guidelines/diagnosis-and-management-of-work-related-mental-he; Harvey, S.B., Modini, M., Joyce, S., et al., 2017, 'Can work make you mentally ill? A systematic meta-review of work-related risk factors for common mental health problems', in *Occup Environ Med*; 74:301–310

17 Workplace Mental Health Institute, *'Mental Health First Aid Australia'*

18 Beyond Blue, *Annual Report 2004–2005*

19 Beyond Blue, 'Beyond Blue offers Australian businesses heavily-subsidised mental health workplace training', (media release)

20 Rajgopal, T., 2010, 'Mental Well-Being At The Workplace', in *Indian Journal Of Occupational And Environmental Medicine* 14 (3): 63. doi:10.4103/0019-5278.75691. https://www.ncbi.nlm.nih.gov/pmc/articles/PMC3062016

21 Australian College of Applied Professions, 'Do Australian organisations really make it OK to bring your whole self to work?', https://www.acap.edu.au/news-and-opinion/do-australian-organisations-really-make-it-ok-to-bring-your-whole-self-to-work accessed 8 Jan 2023

22 Black Dog Institute. 'Black Dog The changing world of work and its impact on Australians' mental health' https://www.blackdoginstitute.org.au/news/the-changing-world-of-work-and-its-impact-on-australians-mental-health/ (Recommendations for Government: Strengthen protections for workers through industrial relations laws to mitigate the effects of insecure work, casualisation, and the gig economy on mental health.)

23 Harvey, et al., *'Work and depression/anxiety disorders'*, 17–18

24 ABS, '6362.0 – Employer Training Expenditure and Practices'

25 Mental Health First Aid Australia, accessed 7 July 2019; Mental Health First Aid International, http://www.mhfainternational.org/; Mental Health First Aid USA, 'Mental Health First Aid for Workplace'; https://www.mentalhealthfirstaid.org/population-focused-modules/workplace/, Mental Health at Work, 'Workplace training', https://www.mentalhealthatwork.org.uk/resource/workplace-training/?read=more, Mental Health America, 'Workplace Training', https://www.mentalhealthamerica.net/workplace-training-and-resources, Mental Health Works, http://www.mentalhealthworks.ca/who-we-are

26 Jaman, P., and Staglin, G.K., 2019, It's time to end the stigma around mental health in the workplace, World Economic Forum. https://www.weforum.org/agenda/2019/05/its-time-to-end-the-stigma-around-mental-health-in-the-workplace

27 Dorter, J., 2019, *The impact of Psychosocial factors on Mental Health and their implications in Life Insurance*; Safe Work Australia, 'Mental Health'; Safe Work Australia, *Work-related psychological health and safety: A systematic approach to meeting your duties*; MLC Life Insurance, 'Dealing with depression and anxiety'; AMA, *Mental illness and life insurance*; headspace, 'How to get al mental health care plan'; Mazza, et al., *Clinical guideline for the diagnosis and management of work-related mental health conditions in general practice*; RACGP, 'Evidence to guide and support GPs'; Harvey, et al., *Work and depression/anxiety disorders*; ibid.

28 AIHW, *Australia's children*, Canberra, AIHW, 2020, https://www.aihw.gov.au/reports/children-youth/australias-children/contents/health/children-mental-illness; Tuohy, W., '"Shocking" numbers of children presenting with mental health issues' in *Sydney Morning Herald*, 24 January 2021, https://www.smh.com.au/national/shocking-numbers-of-children-presenting-with-mental-health-issues-20210123-p56wbp.html; Whitely, *Overprescribing Madness*

29 TAL, 'Our partners', https://www.tal.com.au/about-us/our-commitments/our-partners

30 Industry SuperFunds, 'Income protection insurance', https://www.industrysuper.com/understand-super/insurance-in-super/income-protection-insurance

31 Dorter, J., 2019, *The impact of Psychosocial factors on Mental Health and their implications in Life Insurance*, KPMG

32 AIHW, *Australia's Health 2016*, Canberra: AIHW, 13 September 2016, https://www.aihw.gov.au/reports/australias-health/australias-health-2016/contents/summary

33 Raven, M., 2019, 'Workplace mental health: a strategic driver of overdiagnosis', *BMJ Evidence-Based Medicine* 24: A62–A63, https://ebm.bmj.com/content/24/Suppl_2/A62.2

34 Dorter, J., 2019, *The impact of Psychosocial factors on Mental Health and their implications in Life Insurance*

35 KPMG, , 2013, *The economic cost of suicide in Australia*, Canberra: Menslink, https://menslink.org.au/wp-content/uploads/2013/10/KPMG-Economic-cost-of-suicide-in-Australia-Menslink.pdf; Cook, L., *'Mental health in Australia: a quick guide'*, Canberra: Commonwealth of Australia, 14 February 2019 https://www.aph.gov.au/About_Parliament/Parliamentary_Departments/Parliamentary_Library/pubs/rp/rp1819/Quick_Guides/MentalHealth

36 Safe Work Australia, 'Mental Health'

37 Safe Work Australia, *Work Related Mental Disorders Profile (2015)* https://www.safeworkaustralia.gov.au/system/files/documents/1702/work-related-mental-disorders-profile.pdf

38 Dorter, J., 2019, *The impact of Psychosocial factors on Mental Health and their implications in Life Insurance*

39 Safe Work Australia, 'Mental Health'

40 Berry, S., 'Why we need to hear about our boss' mental health' in *Sydney Morning Herald*, 11 September 2019, https://www.smh.com.au/lifestyle/health-and-wellness/why-we-need-to-hear-about-our-boss-mental-health-20190910-p52ptl.html

41 Bezborodovs and Thornicroft, 'Stigmatisation of mental illness in the workplace'

42 Australian Government Department of Social Services, *Disability Support Pension (DSP) June* 2016 (Canberra: Commonwealth of Australia, 2016), https://data.gov.au/data/dataset/4ccff587-4a46-4ab9-8833-76dadaa10ebe/resource/b6c50479-ffce-4d12-9fe2-afef7b2282c7/download/disability-support-pension-payment-trends-and-profile-report-june-2016.pdf

43 Victoria Legal Aid, 'Disability support pension checklist', updated 30 August 2021, https://www.legalaid.vic.gov.au/find-legal-answers/centrelink/disability-support-pension#checklist

44 Australian Government Department of Social Services, 'Social Security Guide: 3.6.3.50 Guidelines to Table 5 – Mental Health Function', reviewed 10 May 2021, https://guides.dss.gov.au/guide-social-security-law/3/6/3/50

45 ibid.

46 Human Rights Commission, 'Workers with Mental Illness: a Practical Guide for Managers', https://humanrights.gov.au/sites/default/files/document/publication/workers_mental_illness_guide_0.pdf

47 Baum, G., 'Mental health emphasis "overcooked"', *Age*, 27 February 2019, https://www.theage.com.au/sport/afl/mental-health-emphasis-overcooked-20190227-p510on.html

48 'Suicide: Facts and Myths', Square, https://www.square.org.au Introduction

49 Life Insurance Industry, *Life Insurance Industry Response To: Productivity Commission's Draft Report on the Social & Economic Benefits of Improving Mental Health*, 72; 75

50 Dorter, J., 2019, *The impact of Psychosocial factors on Mental Health and their implications in Life Insurance*; 48; Australian Government Department of Social Services, 'Understanding mental health in your workplace', https://www.jobaccess.gov.au/employers/understanding-mental-health-your-workplace; SANE Australia, 'Mental illness & the workplace: How to help', https://www.sane.org/information-stories/facts-and-guides/mental-illness-and-the-workplace#how-to-help; Worklogic, 'Are You OK? Wellbeing, Performance and Conduct of Employees with a Mental Illness', https://www.worklogic.com.au/whistleblower-reporting-service/

are-you-ok-wellbeing-performance-and-conduct-of-employees-with-a-mental-illness/; NB Lawyers, 'Managing Mental Illness In The Workplace', 28 September 2021,https:// www.lawyersforemployers.com.au/managing-mental-illness-in-the-workplace

51 Worklogic, *Are You OK? Wellbeing, Performance and Conduct of Employees with a Mental Illness*

52 Dorter, J., 2019, *The impact of Psychosocial factors on Mental Health and their implications in Life Insurance*

53 ibid., 25

54 Life Insurance Industry, *Life Insurance Industry Response To: Productivity Commission's Draft Report on the Social & Economic Benefits of Improving Mental Health*

55 Summerfield, D., 2013, '"Global mental health" is an oxymoron and medical imperialism' in *BMJ* 346, no. f3509, doi: 10.1136/bmj.f3509; Summerfield, D., 2012, 'The exaggerated claims of the mental health industry' in *BMJ* 344, no. e1791, doi: https://doi.org/10.1136/bmj.e1791; Summerfield, D., 2008, 'How scientifically valid is the knowledge base of global mental health?' in *BMJ* 336): 992–994; Bemme, D., and D'souza, N., 2014, 'Global mental health and its discontents: An inquiry into the making of global and local scale' in *Transcultural Psychiatry* 51, no. 6: 850–874, doi: 10.1177/1363461514539830 doi: https://doi.org/10.1136/bmj.39513.441030.AD; http:// somatosphere.net/2012/global-mental-health-and-its-discontents.html/; Fernando, S., 2011, 'A "global" mental health program or markets for Big Pharma?' in *Open Mind* 168: 2353–2353; Robert Whitaker, 2010, *Anatomy of an epidemic*, New York: Crown; Mills, C., 2014, *Decolonizing global mental health,* London: Routledge; International Mental Health Collaborating Network, 'Critical and post psychiatry', https://imhcn. org/bibliography/transforming-services/critical-psychiatry

56 WHO, 'Mental health in the workplace', https://www.who.int/ teams/mental-health-and-substance-use/promotion-prevention/ mental-health-in-the-workplace

57 Leka, S., Griffiths, and Cox, T., 2003, *Work organisation and stress : systematic problem approaches for employers, managers and trade union representatives,* Geneva: WHO https://www.who.int/occupational_health/publications/en/oehstress.pdf

58 Dembe, et al., 'Inpatient hospital care for work-related injuries and illnesses'

59 Mazza, D., et al., 2015, 'General practitioners and sickness certification for injury in Australia' in *BMC Family Practice* 16, no. 1, DOI 10.1186/s12875-015-0307-9

60 RACGP, *General Practice: Health of the Nation 2018*, Harvey, et al., 'Is the prevalence of mental illness increasing in Australia?'

61 Knudsen, A.K., Øverland, S., Aakvaag, H.F., et al., 2010, 'Common mental disorders and disability pension award: Seven year follow-up of the HUSK study' in *Journal of Psychosomatic Research* 69, no.1: 59–67, doi:10.1016/j.jpsychores.2010.03.007

62 Letrilliart, l., and Barrau, A., 2012, 'Difficulties with the sickness certification process in general practice and possible solutions: A systematic review' in *European Journal of General Practice* 18, no. 4: 219–228, DOI:10.3109/13814788.2012.727795; Mazza, et al., 'General practitioners and sickness certification for injury in Australia'; Brijnath, B., et al., 2016, 'Is clinician refusal to treat an emerging problem in injury compensation systems?' in *BMJ Open* 6, no. 1: 3, DOI: 10.1136/bmjopen-2015-009423

63 Brijnath, et al., 'Is clinician refusal to treat an emerging problem in injury compensation systems?'

Chapter 5 – Under pressure: the role of general medical practice

1 Commonwealth of Australia, 2006, 'Access to mental health services', in *A national approach to mental health – from crisis to community First Report,* Canberra, https:// www.aph.gov.au/Parliamentary_Business/Committees/Senate/Former_Committees/ mentalhealth/report/c06.

2   AIHW, 2016, *Mental health services—in brief 2016. Cat. no. HSE 180*, Canberra: AIHW, https://www.aihw.gov.au/getmedia/681f0689-8360-4116-b1cc-9d2276b65703/20299. pdf.aspx?inline=true

3   RACGP, *General Practice: Health of the Nation 2018*; AIHW, *Mental health services— in brief 2019*; AIHW, *Mental health services in Australia: Mental health-related prescriptions*

4   AIHW, *Mental health services—in brief 2019*

5   ibid.

6   AIHW, *Mental health-related services provided by general practitioners*, updated October 2018 https://www.aihw.gov.au/getmedia/9fe70a73-e1c5-4139-8f3b-12f144c663d9/Mental-health-services-provided-by-general-practitioners.pdf.aspx

7   Plaskitt, A., 'It's rare to be able to tell the truth – here's what's wrong with Australia's mental health system', in *Guardian*, 26 April 2021, https://www.theguardian.com/australia-news/2021/apr/26/its-rare-to-be-able-to-tell-the-truth-heres-whats-wrong-with-the-mental-health-system

8   RACGP, 'DH16 – Doctors' health contextual unit'; Cohen and Rhydderch, 'Measuring a doctor's performance'; Elliot, Tan and Norris, *The mental health of doctors*

9   RACGP, *General Practice: Health of the Nation 2018*; AMA, 'Health and wellbeing of doctors and medical students – 2020'

10   Brown, G.W., et al., 2010, 'Antidepressants, social adversity and outcome of depression in general practice', in *Journal of Affective Disorders* 121, no. 3: 239–246, doi: 10.1016/j.jad.2009.06.004

11   Dowrick and Frances, 'Medicalising unhappiness'

12   ibid.

13   Kirk and Kutchkins, 'The myth of reliability of DSM'

14   Dowrick and Frances, 'Medicalising unhappiness'

15   Brown, et al., 'Antidepressants, social adversity and outcome of depression in general practice'

16   Fleury, M-J., Imboua, A., Aubé, D., et al., 2012, 'General practitioners' management of mental disorders: a rewarding practice with considerable obstacles', in *BMC Family Practice* 13, no. 19, doi:10.1186/1471-2296-13-19

17   RACGP, *General Practice: Health of the Nation 2018*

18   Cosgrove, L., Erlich, D., and Shaughnessy, A.F., 2019, 'No Magic Pill: A Prescription for Enhanced Shared Decision-Making for Depression Treatment', in *The Journal of the American Board of Family Medicine* 32, no. 1: 6–9, doi: 10.3122/jabfm.2019.01.180182

19   Davidsen, A.S., and Fosgerau, C.F., 2014, 'What is depression? Psychiatrists' and GPs' experiences of diagnosis and the diagnostic process', in *International Journal of Qualitative Studies on Health and Well-being* 9, no. 1, doi:10.3402/qhw.v9.24866

20   Fleury, et al., 'General practitioners' management of mental disorders'; Irving, G., Neves, A.L., Dambha-Miller, H., et al., 2017, 'International variations in primary care physician consultation time: a systematic review of 67 countries', in *BMJ Open* 7, no. 10, doi: 10.1136/bmjopen-2017-017902; Buckman, L., and Griffiths, M., 'Should GPs' daily number of consultations be capped?' in *BMJ* 361 (2018), doi: 10.1136/bmj.k1947

21   AMA, 'Health and wellbeing of doctors and medical students – 2020'; Cohen and Rhydderch, 'Measuring a doctor's performance'

22   Hengartner, 'Methodological flaws, conflicts of interest, and scientific fallacies'; Hengartner and Plöderl, 'Statistically significant antidepressant-placebo differences on subjective symptom-rating scales do not prove that the drugs work'

23   Royal College of Psychiatrists, May 2019, *Position statement on antidepressants and depression*, https://www.rcpsych.ac.uk/docs/default-source/improving-care/better-mh-policy/position-statements/ps04_19—-antidepressants-and-depression.pdf?sfvrsn=ddea9473_5

24 Cleary, B., 'Daddy, please kill me I can't do this any more': Meet the CHILDREN prescribed anti-depressants for anxiety that "made them suicidal" – as scores of parents join in a class action', in *Daily Mail Australia*, 23 April 2017, https://www.dailymail.co.uk/news/article-4431472/Anti-depressants-caused-suicidal-thoughts-children.html; Ison, S., 'Aged Just Seven, My Girl Became Death-Obsessed', in *West Australian*, 27 June 2019, http://enewspaper2.smedia.com.au/wandaily/shared/ShowArticle.aspx?doc=WAN%2F2019%2F06%2F27&entity=Ar01001&sk=72AD3E36&fbclid=IwAR3DC4NN2vONwtD0f4GMHIiEWnct-lOvuxYiLy7gypjhqdD2oHXQ4YUAM_4;

25 US Food and Drug Administration, *Revisions to Product Labeling*, accessed 19 July 2019, https://www.fda.gov/media/77404/download.

26 Bielefeldt, A.Ø., Danborg, P.B. and Gøtzsche, P.C., 2016, 'Precursors to suicidality and violence on antidepressants: systematic review of trials in adult healthy volunteers', in *Journal of the Royal Society of Medicine* 109, no. 10: 381–392. doi:10.1177/0141076816666805; Adshead, G., 2017, 'Antidepressants and murder: case not closed', in *BMJ* 358, no. j3697, doi: 10.1136/bmj.j3697; Davies and Read, 'A systematic review into the incidence, severity and duration of antidepressant withdrawal effects'; FDA, *Revisions to Product Labeling*

27 Hengartner and Plöderl, 'False Beliefs in Academic Psychiatry'

28 Davies and Read, 'A systematic review into the incidence, severity and duration of antidepressant withdrawal effects'; Bielefeldt, Danborg and Gøtzsche, 'Precursors to suicidality and violence on antidepressants'; Royal College of Psychiatrists, *Position statement on antidepressants and depression*

Chapter 6 – Medicating human distress: effectiveness and harms from antidepressants

1 Whitely, *Overprescribing Madness*, 12

2 Hengartner, M., and Plöderl, M., 2018, 'False Beliefs in Academic Psychiatry: The Case of Antidepressant Drugs', in *Ethical Human Psychology and Psychiatry* 20, no.1: 6–16, doi: 10.1891/1559-4343.20.1.6; Davies and Read, 'A systematic review into the incidence, severity and duration of antidepressant withdrawal effects'; Cartwright, C., Gibson, K., Read, J., et al., 'Long-term antidepressant use: patient perspectives of benefits and adverse effects', in *Patient preference and adherence* 10 (2016): 1401–1407, doi:10.2147/PPA.S110632

3 Chouinard, G., and Chouinard, V-A., 2015, 'New Classification of Selective Serotonin Reuptake Inhibitor Withdrawal', in *Psychotherapy and Psychosomatics* 84, 63–71, doi: 10.1159/000371865; Andrews, P., 'Things Your Doctor Should Tell You About Antidepressants', in *Mad in America*, 12 September 2012, http://www.madinamerica.com/2012/09/things-your-doctor-should-tell-you-about-antidepressants/; Hengartner and Plöderl, 'False Beliefs in Academic Psychiatry'; Davies and Read, 'A systematic review into the incidence, severity and duration of antidepressant withdrawal effects'; Cartwright, et al., 'Long-term antidepressant use'

4 OECD, *Health at a Glance 2017: OECD Indicators* (Paris: OECD Publishing, 2017), https://doi.org/10.1787/health_glance-2017-en; Australian Institute of Health and Welfare, *Australia's Health 2008* (Canberra: AIHW, 2008), https://www.aihw.gov.au/getmedia/106ff693-72d0-4fd5-98d9-24259254d77f/ah08.pdf.aspx?inline=true; Australian Government Department of Health and Ageing, *Australian Statistics on Medicines 2006* (Canberra: Commonwealth of Australia, 2006), https://www.pbs.gov.au/info/statistics/asm/asm-2006; Australian Government Department of Health and Ageing, *Australian Statistics on Medicines 2003* (Canberra: Commonwealth of Australia, 2005), https://www.pbs.gov.au/info/statistics/asm/asm-2003; Australian Government Department of Health. '2019–20 Federal Budget advances long term national health plan'

(Canberra: Commonwealth of Australia, 2 April 2019), https://www.health.gov.au/news/2019-20-federal-budget-advances-long-term-national-health-plan

5   OECD, *Health at a Glance 2017*, 'Pharmaceutical consumption'

6   Gould. S. and Friedman L.F., 2016, 'Something startling is going on with antidepressant use around the world', in *Business Insider*, https://www.businessinsider.com/countries-largest-antidepressant-drug-users-2016-2?r=AU&IR=T

7   Pratt, L., Brody, D., and Gu, Q., 2017, *'Antidepressant use among persons aged 12 and over: United States, 2011–2014'*, Hyattsville, Maryland: National Center for Health Statistics https://www.cdc.gov/nchs/products/databriefs/db283.htm

8   Gould and Friedman, 'Something startling is going on with antidepressant use around the world'

9   Iacobucci, G., 2019, 'NHS prescribed record number of antidepressants last year', in *British Medical Journal* 364:l1508, https://doi.org/10.1136/bmj.l1508

10   Gould and Friedman, 'Something startling is going on with antidepressant use around the world'

11   OECD, *OECD Health Statistics: Pharmaceutical market* (Paris, OECD, 2021), https://doi.org/10.1787/health-data-en

12   AIHW, Mental health services in Australia https://www.aihw.gov.au/reports/mental-health-services/mental-health-services-in-australia/report-contents/mental-health-related-prescriptions, accessed 9 Oct 2022

13   ibid.

14   Westbury, J., Gee, P., Ling, T. et al., 2018, 'More action needed: Psychotropic prescribing in Australian residential aged care', in *Australian & New Zealand Journal Of Psychiatry* 53, no. 2: 136–147, doi: 10.1177/0004867418758919

15   Erken, N., Kaya, D., Dost, F., et al., 2022, 'Antidepressant-induced serotonin syndrome in older patients: a cross-sectional study', in *Psychogeriatrics,* 22(4), 502–508. DOI: 10.1111/psyg.12849

16   Harrison, S., Sluggett, J., Lang, C., et al., 2020, 'The dispensing of psychotropic medicines to older people before and after they enter residential aged care' in *Medical Journal of Australia,* 212(7), 309–313

17   Cuijpers, P., Stringaris, A., and Wolpert, M., 2020, 'Treatment outcomes for depression: challenges and opportunities', in *Lancet Psychiatry* 7, no. 11: 925–927, doi: 10.1016/s2215-0366 (20)30036-5; Maslej, M.M., Furukawa, T.A., Cipriani, A., et al., 'Individual differences in response to antidepressants: A meta-analysis of placebo-controlled randomized clinical trials', in *JAMA Psychiatry* 78, no. 5 (2021): 490–497, doi:10.1001/JAMA psychiatry.2020.4564

18   Kirsch, I., 2019, 'Placebo Effect in the Treatment of Depression and Anxiety', in *Frontiers in Psychiatry* 10 (2019), doi: 10.3389/fpsyt.2019.00407; Oronowicz-Jaśkowiak, W., and Bąbel, P., 2019, 'Twenty years after "Listening to Prozac but hearing placebo". Do we hear placebo even louder?', in *Health Psychology Review* 7, no. 1: 1–8, DOI: 10.5114/hpr.2019.83383; Hengartner, M., and Plöderl, M., 2019, 'What are the chances for personalised treatment with antidepressants? Detection of patient-by-treatment interaction with a variance ratio meta-analysis', in *BMJ Open* 9 (2019), doi: 10.1136/bmjopen-2019-034816

19   Kirsch, I., Deacon, B., Huedo-Medina, T.B., et al., 2008, 'Initial Severity and Antidepressant Benefits: A Meta-Analysis of Data Submitted to the Food and Drug Administration' in *Plos Medicine* 5, no. 2. doi: 10.1371/journal.pmed.0050044

20   Moncrieff, J., Cooper, R., and Stockmann, T., et al, 2022, 'The serotonin theory of depression: a systematic umbrella review of the evidence', in *Molecular Psychiatry*, https://www.nature.com/articles/s41380-022-01661-0

21   Turner, et al., 'Selective Publication of Antidepressant Trials and Its Influence on Apparent Efficacy'

22   OECD, 'Antidepressant drugs consumption, 2000 and 2015 (or nearest year)' in *Health at a Glance 2017* https://www.oecd-ilibrary.org/social-issues-migration-health/health-at-a-glance-2017/antidepressant-drugs-consumption-2000-and-2015-or-nearest-year_health_glance-2017-graph181-en; Mordor Intelligence, 'Antidepressant Market – Growth, Trends, and Forecast (2019–2024)', accessed 6 August 2019, https://www.mordorintelligence.com/industry-reports/antidepressants-market

23   Davies and Read, 'A systematic review into the incidence, severity and duration of antidepressant withdrawal effects'; FDA, *Revisions to Product Labeling*; Hengartner, M., and Plöderl, M.,2019, 'Newer-Generation Antidepressants and Suicide Risk in Randomized Controlled Trials: A Re-Analysis of the FDA Database', in *Psychotherapy and Psychosomatics* 88, no. 4: 247–248, doi: 10.1159/000501215; Hengartner and Plöderl, 'False Beliefs in Academic Psychiatry'; Bielefeldt, Danborg and Gøtzsche, 'Precursors to suicidality and violence on antidepressants'; Royal College of Psychiatrists, *Position statement on antidepressants and depression*; Gøtzsche, P.C., Young, A.H., and Crace, J., 2015, 'Does long-term use of psychiatric drugs cause more harm than good?', in *BMJ* 350, doi: 10.1136/bmj.h2435; Whitaker, *Anatomy of an epidemic*; Breggin, P.R., *Medication madness* (New York: St Martin's Griffin, 2008); Healy, D., Herxheimer, and Menkes, D.B., 2006, 'Antidepressants and Violence: Problems at the Interface of Medicine and Law', in *Plos Medicine* 3, no. 9, https://doi.org/10.1371/journal.pmed.0030372; Maslej, M.M., Bolker, B.M., Russell, M.J., et al., 2017, 'The Mortality and Myocardial Effects of Antidepressants Are Moderated by Pre-existing Cardiovascular Disease: A Meta-Analysis', in *Psychotherapy and Psychosomatics* 86, no. 5: 268–282, doi: 10.1159/000477940; Harvard School of Health, 'What are the real risks of antidepressants?', 17 August 2021, https://www.health.harvard.edu/newsletter_article/what-are-the-real-risks-of-antidepressants; Evans, E.A., and Sullivan, M.A., 2014, 'Abuse and misuse of antidepressants', *Substance abuse and rehabilitation* 5: 107–120, doi:10.2147/SAR.S37917; Haddad, P.M., 2005, 'Do antidepressants cause dependence?' in *Epidemiologia E Psichiatria Sociale* 14, no. 2: 58–62. doi:10.1017/S1121189X00006254

24   Jureidini, J., 2016, 'Antidepressants fail, but no cause for therapeutic gloom' in *Lancet*, 388. 10.1016/S0140-6736(16)30585-2

25   Aubusson, K., 'Antidepressants ineffective and harmful for children and teens, major review finds' in *Sydney Morning Herald,* 9 June 2016, https://www.smh.com.au/healthcare/antidepressants-ineffective-and-harmful-for-children-and-teens-major-review-finds-20160609-gpezxx.html

26   FDA, *Revisions to Product Labeling* https://www.fda.gov/media/77404/download accessed 19 July 2019

27   Whitely, M., Raven, M. and Jureidini, J., 2020, 'Antidepressant prescribing and suicide/self-harm by Young Australians: Regulatory warnings, contradictory advice, and long-term trends' in *Frontiers in Psychiatry*, 11 https://doi.org/10.3389/fpsyt.2020.00478

28   Anderson, K., Lind, J.N., Simeone, R.M., et al., 2020, 'Maternal Use of Specific Antidepressant Medications During Early Pregnancy and the Risk of Selected Birth Defects' in *JAMA Psychiatry* 77, no. 12: 1246–1255, doi:10.1001/jamapsychiatry.2020.2453

29   FDA, *Revisions to Product Labeling*; Gøtzsche, P.C., 2016, 'Antidepressants are addictive and increase the risk of relapse', *BMJ* 352, doi: 10.1136/bmj.i574; Bielefeldt, Danborg and Gøtzsche, 'Precursors to suicidality and violence on antidepressants'; Healy, Herxheimer and Menkes, 'Antidepressants and Violence'

30   Beyond Blue, 'Tackling back-to-school anxiety', https://healthyfamilies.beyondblue.org.au/age-6-12/mental-health-conditions-in-children/anxiety/tackling-back-to-school-anxiety, Beyond Blue, 'Seeking support for your child', https://healthyfamilies.beyondblue.org.au/age-1-5/seeking-support-for-your-child, Beyond Blue, 'Anxiety', https://beyou.edu.au/fact-sheets/mental-health-issues-and-conditions/anxiety; Beyond Blue, 'Beyond Blue Chair The Hon Julia Gillard,

AC, launches "Be You", Beyond Blue, https://www.beyondblue.org.au/media/
news/news/2018/10/31/beyond-blue-chair-julia-gillard-launches-be-you 'Children
(aged 0–12), https://www.beyondblue.org.au/who-does-it-affect/children, From
August 2018, Beyond Blue will lead a new National Education Initiative with
support from headspace and Early Childhood Australia, with funding from the
Australian Government Department of Health', https://thesector.com.au/2018/10/09/
beyondblue-launches-new-national-education-initiative/

31   Beyond Blue, 2015, *Victoria's next 10-year mental health strategy – Discussion paper*,
      Hawthorn West: Beyond Blue, https://www.beyondblue.org.au/docs/default-source/
      about-beyond-blue/policy-submissions/victoria's-next-10-year-mental-health-
      strategy_beyondblue-submission.pdf?sfvrsn=e4aa49ea_2
32   FDA, *Revisions to Product Labeling*
33   Hengartner and Plöderl, 'Newer-Generation Antidepressants and Suicide Risk in
      Randomized Controlled Trials'
34   Hengartner and Plöderl, 'Newer-Generation Antidepressants and Suicide Risk in
      Randomized Controlled Trials'; Bielefeldt, Danborg and Gøtzsche, 'Precursors to
      suicidality and violence on antidepressants'; Gøtzsche, Young and Crace, 'Does long-
      term use of psychiatric drugs cause more harm than good?'; Breggin, *Medication
      madness*; Healy, Herxheimer and Menkes, 'Antidepressants and Violence'; Maslej, et
      al., 'The Mortality and Myocardial Effects of Antidepressants Are Moderated by Pre-
      existing Cardiovascular Disease'
35   Gøtzsche, P., 2017, 'Antidepressants increase the risk of suicide, violence and
      homicide at all ages', in *BMJ* https://www.bmj.com/content/358/bmj.j3697/rr-4
      (Accessed 22 July 2019)
36   Healy, D., 2017, 'Antidepressants and murder: justice denied' in *BMJ*; 358 doi: https://
      doi.org/10.1136/bmj.j4196, 26 September 2017
37   PR Newswire, 'Mental Health Watchdog Says UK TV Documentary
      "Prescription for Murder?" Should Prompt U.S. Investigations Into
      Psychotropic Drug Violence', https://www.prnewswire.com/news-releases/
      mental-health-watchdog-says-uk-tv-documentary-prescription-for-murder-should-
      prompt-us-investigations-into-psychotropic-drug-violence-300498170.htm accessed
      11 Jan 2023
38   Citizens Commission on Human Rights, Psychiatric Drugs: Create Violence &
      Suicide https://www.cchrint.org/pdfs/violence-report.pdf
39   Davies and Read, 'A systematic review into the incidence, severity and duration of
      antidepressant withdrawal effects'
40   Royal College of Psychiatrists, 'Antidepressants: Do antidepressants have side-
      effects?', accessed 2 May 2021, https://www.rcpsych.ac.uk/mental-health/
      treatments-and-wellbeing/antidepressants; NHS, 'Side effects – Antidepressants',
      https://www.nhs.uk/mental-health/talking-therapies-medicine-treatments/
      medicines-and-psychiatry/antidepressants/side-effects
41   Chouinard, G., Annable, L., and Bradwejn, J., 1984, 'An early phase II clinical trial
      of tomoxetine (LY139603) in the treatment of newly admitted depressed patients' in
      Psychopharmacology 83, no. 1: 126–8, DOI:10.1007/BF00427436
42   'Adverse events information related to Strattera obtained from the Therapeutic
      Goods Administration' Public Case Detail reports, referenced in Whitely, M.,
      Overprescribing Madness, 253
43   Lesley Ashmall, 'The "extreme" side-effects of antidepressants' in *BBC News*, 19
      October 2016, https://www.bbc.com/news/health-37682355; See the following
      Facebook groups for individual accounts of harm from antidepressants:
      Australian Antidepressants Awareness: https://www.facebook.com/
          AustralianAntidepressantClassAction
      Do No Harm: https://www.facebook.com/groups/DoNoHarmGroup

Cymbalta Dangers International: https://www.facebook.com/
CymbaltaDangersInternational

Psychiatric Drugs Book Collaboration: https://www.facebook.com/groups/Breakin
gFreeFromPsychiatricDrugs/?source_id=527725173994669

Speak Out Against Psychiatry: https://www.facebook.com/groups/speakoutagainst
psychiatry/?source_id=527725173994669

Psychiatric Drugs Destroy Life: https://www.facebook.com/
groups/12507837106/?source_id=527725173994669

International lawsuit against coercive psychiatry: https://www.facebook.com/
groups/1631567377147931/?source_id=527725173994669

Let's Talk Withdrawal: https://www.facebook.com/groups/LetsTalkWithdrawal

Antidepressant-Induced Cravings for Alcohol: https://www.facebook.com/
groups/1688062138113514

Cured to Death: Pharmaceutical Injury Stories: https://www.facebook.com/
groups/2654699238186454

Paxil (Paroxetine, Seroxat) Should Be Illegal: https://www.facebook.com/
groups/370289153168180

Remeron (Mirtazapine) Should Be Illegal: https://www.facebook.com/groups/
RemeronandMirtazapine

Psych Med Withdrawal Syndrome Support Group: https://www.facebook.com/
groups/126400127922735

Tardive Dyskinesia/Akathisia Support Group: https://www.facebook.com/
groups/1651647445098837

Breaking Free From Psychiatric Drugs Book Collaboration: https://www.facebook.
com/groups/BreakingFreeFromPsychiatricDrugs

Abilify (Aripiprazole) Should Be Illegal: https://www.facebook.com/
groups/1082455861794780

SSRIs/Antidepressants Withdrawal (Paroxetine, Paxil, Seroxat): https://www.
facebook.com/groups/204732929546136

AKATHISIA ALLIANCE for Education and Research: https://www.facebook.com/
groups/akathisiaalliance

Risperdal (Risperidone) Should Be Illegal: https://www.facebook.com/
groups/818693634915069

Damaged by Psychiatry: https://www.facebook.com/groups/966428756862718

44   *Herald Sun*, 'Time To Wean Kids Off Drugs', 27 June 2022 https://
www.heraldsun.com.au/subscribe/news/1/?sourceCode=HSWEB_
WRE170_a_GGL&dest=https%3A%2F%2Fwww.heraldsun.com.
au%2Fnews%2Fnational%2Fnew-tga-review-as-number-of-children-prescribed-
antidepressants-doubles-in-10-years%2Fnews-story%2Fd1f69f4f6a501ef4f150db9-
8d934f1b7&memtype=anonymous&mode=premium&v21=dyn
amic-high-control-score&V21spcbehaviour=append
Mr Butler has asked his department to review prescribing of the drugs and develop
new evidence-based guidelines for their safe use

45   Davies and Read, 'A systematic review into the incidence, severity and duration of
antidepressant withdrawal effects'

46   Royal College of Psychiatrists, *Position statement on antidepressants and depression*

47   Davey, 'Urgent need to find safe ways for patients to withdraw from antidepressants'

48   Van Leeuwen, E., van Driel, M.L., Horowitz, M.A., et al., 2021, 'Approaches for
discontinuation versus continuation of long-term antidepressant use for depressive
and anxiety disorders in adults' in Cochrane Database of Systematic Reviews,
2021(4). Available at: https://doi.org/10.1002/14651858.cd013495.pub2

49 Guy, A., Brown, M., Lewis, S., et al., 2020, 'The "patient voice": patients who experience antidepressant withdrawal symptoms are often dismissed, or misdiagnosed with relapse, or a new medical condition' in *Ther Adv Psychopharmacol*, 10:2045125320967183. doi: 10.1177/2045125320967183; Stone, J., Burton, C. and Carson, A., 2021, 'Recognising and explaining functional neurological disorder' in BMJ 371, doi: 10.1136/bmj.m3745; Brown, M., and Lewis, S., 2021, 'The patient voice: Antidepressant withdrawal, medically unexplained symptoms and functional neurological disorders' in *Journal of Critical Psychology, Counselling and Psychotherapy* 20, no. 4: 14–20; Chouinard and Chouinard, 'New Classification of Selective Serotonin Reuptake Inhibitor Withdrawal'; Gøtzsche, P., 'Is Psychiatry Evidence Based?', Part 2, Ch. 2, from *Mental Health Survival Kit and Withdrawal from Psychiatric Drugs*, Mad in America, 8 March 2021, https://www.madinamerica.com/2021/03/mental-health-survival-kit-chapter-2-part-2/; Healy, *Let Them Eat Prozac*.

50 Royal College of Psychiatrists, 'Stopping antidepressants', accessed 18 May 2021, https://www.rcpsych.ac.uk/mental-health/treatments-and-wellbeing/stopping-antidepressants?searchTerms=stopping%20antidepressants

51 Malhi, G.S., et al., 2015, 'Royal Australian New Zealand College of Psychiatrists clinical practice guidelines for mood disorders, https://www.ranzcp.org/files/resources/college_statements/clinician/cpg/mood-disorders-cpg.aspx, *Australian and New Zealand Journal of Psychiatry* 49, no. 12 (2015):1–185

52 ibid., 31–32

53 Malhi, et al., *Royal Australian New Zealand College of Psychiatrists clinical practice guidelines for mood disorders*, 37–38

54 Harvard School of Health, 'What are the real risks of antidepressants?'; Evans and Sullivan, 'Abuse and misuse of antidepressants'; Haddad, 'Do antidepressants cause dependence?'; Gøtzsche, 'Antidepressants are addictive and increase the risk of relapse'; Harriet Fraad, 'Profiting from mental ill-health', in *Guardian*, 16 March 2011, https://www.theguardian.com/commentisfree/cifamerica/2011/mar/15/psychology-healthcare

55 Jelinek, G., and Neate, S., 2009, 'The influence of the pharmaceutical industry in medicine' in *Journal of Law and Medicine* 17, 216–23; Campsall, P., Colizza, K., Strauset, S. et al., 2016, 'Financial Relationships between Organizations That Produce Clinical Practice Guidelines and the Biomedical Industry: A Cross-Sectional Study' in *Plos Medicine* 13, no. 5, 1002029.doi:10.1371/journal.pmed.1002029; Schwartz, L.M., and Woloshin, S., 2019, 'Medical Marketing in the United States, 1997–2016' in *JAMA* 321, no. 1 (2019), doi: 10.1001/jama.2018.19320; Fickweiler, F., Fickweiler, W., and Urbach, E., 2017, 'Interactions between physicians and the pharmaceutical industry generally and sales representatives specifically and their association with physicians' attitudes and prescribing habits: a systematic review' in *BMJ Open* 7, no. 9 , doi: 10.1136/bmjopen-2017-016408; Larkin, I., Ang, D., Steinhart, J., et al., 2017, 'Association Between Academic Medical Center Pharmaceutical Detailing Policies and Physician Prescribing' in *JAMA* 317, no. 17. doi: 10.1001/jama.2017.4039; Kroenke, K., Spitzer, R., and Williams, J., 'The PHQ-9' in *Journal of General Internal Medicine* 16, no. 9 (2001): 606–613, doi: 10.1046/j.1525-1497.2001.016009606.x; Knaus, C., and Evershed, N., 'Pharmaceutical industry donates millions to both Australian political parties', *Guardian*, 25 September 2018, https://www.theguardian.com/business/2018/sep/25/pharmaceutical-industry-donates-millions-to-both-australian-political-parties; Richard Baker, 'Mental health takes industry pills', *Age*, 8 August 2008, https://www.theage.com.au/national/mental-health-takes-industry-pills-20060808-ge2vju.html

56 Fraad, 'Profiting from mental ill-health'

57 Sigler, C., 'Pharma Goes to Court', Faith Seeking Understanding, 29 July 2015, http://faith-seeking-understanding.org/2015/07/29/pharma-goes-to-court/; Frances, A., 2014, *Saving Normal: An Insider's Revolt against Out-of-Control Psychiatric Diagnosis, DSM-5, Big Pharma, and the Medicalization of Ordinary Life*, New York: Harper Collins

Notes

Chapter 7 – The role of the pharmaceutical industry

1 Whitaker, *Anatomy of an epidemic*; Breggin, *Medication madness*; Gøtzsche, Young and Crace, 'Does long-term use of psychiatric drugs cause more harm than good?'; Whitely, *Overprescribing Madness*; Raven, 'Depression and antidepressants in Australia and Beyond'

2 Paykel, 'Basic concepts of depression'

3 Whitely, *Overprescribing Madness*, 18

4 Bulik, B.S., 'The top 10 ad spenders in Big Pharma for 2019' in *FiercePharma*, 19 February 2020 https://www.fiercepharma.com/special-report/top-10-ad-spenders-big-pharma-for-2020.

5 Fortune Business Insights, 'Antidepressants Market Size, Share & COVID-19 Impact Analysis', https://www.fortunebusinessinsights.com/antidepressants-market-105017; IMS Health (Midas), 'U.S. Pharmaceutical Sales – Q4 2013', Drugs.com., updated February 2014, https://www.drugs.com/stats/top100/sales; Matej Mikulik, 'Top 15 pharmaceutical products by sales worldwide 2020', statista, 26 March 2021, https://www.statista.com/statistics/258022/top-10-pharmaceutical-products-by-global-sales-2011 ; Pharmacompass.com., 'Top drugs by sales revenue in 2015: Who sold the biggest blockbuster drugs?', 10 March 2016, https://www.pharmacompass.com/radio-compass-blog/top-drugs-by-sales-revenue-in-2015-who-sold-the-biggest-blockbuster-drugs

6 Fortune Business Insights, 'Antidepressants Market to Touch USD 18.29 Billion by 2027; Growing Awareness about Mental Health Conditions to Fuel the Market', https://www.globenewswire.com/news-release/2021/03/08/2188401/0/en/Antidepressants-Market-to-Touch-USD-18-29-Billion-by-2027-Growing-Awareness-about-Mental-Health-Conditions-to-Fuel-the-Market-Fortune-Business-Insights.html

7 Schwartz and Woloshin, 'Medical Marketing in the United States'

8 Whitely, M., 2014, 'Attention Deficit Hyperactivity Disorder Policy, Practice and Regulatory Capture in Australia 1992–2012', PhD thesis, Curtin University, https://espace.curtin.edu.au

9 Sismondo, S., 2021, 'Epistemic Corruption, the Pharmaceutical Industry, and the Body of Medical Science' in *Front. Res. Metr. Anal.* 6:614013. DOI: 10.3389/frma.2021.614013

10 Jureidini, J., McHenry, L.B., 2022, 'The illusion of evidence-based medicine' in *BMJ* 2022; 376:o702 doi:10.1136/bmj.o702 https://doi.org/10.1136/bmj.o702

11 Jelinek, G., and Neate, S., 2009, 'The influence of the pharmaceutical industry in medicine'; Fabbri, A., Grundy, Q., Mintzeset, B., et al., 2017, 'A cross-sectional analysis of pharmaceutical industry-funded events for health professionals in Australia' in *BMJ Open* 7, doi:10.1136/bmjopen-2017-01670

12 Baker, 'Mental health takes industry pills'; Pfizer, 'Corporate Sponsorships January–December 2012: Mental Health Council of Australia', Pfizer.com.au, 6 August 2018, https://www.pfizer.com.au/corporate-sponsorships-january-december-2012

13 Campsall, et al., 'Financial Relationships between Organizations That Produce Clinical Practice Guidelines and the Biomedical Industry'; Kroenke, Spitzer and Williams, 'The PHQ-9'

14 Horwitz, 'How an age of anxiety became an age of depression'

15 Conrad, P., Slodden, C., 2013, 'The Medicalization of Mental Disorder' in Aneshensel, C.S., Phelan J.C., Bierman, A. (eds) *Handbook of the Sociology of Mental Health,* Handbooks of Sociology and Social Research, Springer, Dordrecht, https://doi.org/10.1007/978-94-007-4276-5_4

16 Greenslit, N.P., and Kaptchuk, T.J., 2012, 'Antidepressants and advertising: psychopharmaceuticals in crisis' in *The Yale Journal of Biology and Medicine* 85, no. 1 (2012): 153–158

17 Horwitz, 'How an age of anxiety became an age of depression'

18 Mintzes, B., Swandari, S., Fabbri, A., et al., 2018, 'Does industry-sponsored education foster overdiagnosis and overtreatment of depression, osteoporosis and over-active bladder syndrome? An Australian cohort study' in *BMJ Open*, 13;8(2):e019027. doi: 10.1136/bmjopen-2017-019027

19 Fickweiler, Fickweiler and Urbach, 'Interactions between physicians and the pharmaceutical industry generally and sales representatives specifically and their association with physicians' attitudes and prescribing habits'; Baker, 'Mental health takes industry pills'; Pfizer, 'Corporate Sponsorships January–December 2012: Mental Health Council of Australia'

20 Larkin, et al., 'Association Between Academic Medical Center Pharmaceutical Detailing Policies and Physician Prescribing'

21 Jelinek and Neate, 'The influence of the pharmaceutical industry in medicine'

22 Campsall, et al., 'Financial Relationships between Organizations That Produce Clinical Practice Guidelines and the Biomedical Industry'

23 ibid.

24 Choudhry, N.K., Stelfox, H.T., and Detsky, A.S., 2002, 'Relationships Between Authors of Clinical Practice Guidelines and the Pharmaceutical Industry' in *JAMA* 287, no. 5: 612–7, doi: 10.1001/jama.287.5.612
    Currie, J., 'The Marketization of Depression: Prescribing SSRI Antidepressants to Women', *Toronto: Women and Health Protection*, May 2005, https://cwhn.ca/en/node/26773

25 Knaus and Evershed, 'Pharmaceutical industry donates millions to both Australian political parties'

26 Baker, 'Mental health takes industry pills'; Pfizer, 'Corporate Sponsorships January–December 2012: Mental Health Council of Australia'

27 Willis, E., and Delbaere, M., 2022, 'Patient Influencers: The Next Frontier in Direct-to-Consumer Pharmaceutical Marketing' in *Journal of Medical Internet Research*, 24(3), p.e29422 https://www.ncbi.nlm.nih.gov/pmc/articles/PMC8924782

Chapter 8 – The language of mental health and the illness paradigm

1 Fried and Nesse, 'Depression sum-scores don't add up'; ABS, *National Survey of Mental Health and Wellbeing: Summary of Results*

2 Paykel, 'Basic concepts of depression'

3 Horwitz, 'How an age of anxiety became an age of depression'

4 King, S., 2020, 'CCHR's Reply to Mental Health Inquiry Commissioner', Citizens Commission on Human Rights, https://cchr.org.au/uncategorized/cchrs-reply-to-mental-health-inquiry-commissioner

5 Safe Work Australia, *Work Related Mental Disorders Profile* (2015), 4

6 Pūras, *Report of the Special Rapporteur on the right of everyone to the enjoyment of the highest attainable standard of physical and mental health*, 3: Point 10; 10: Point 49

7 Scott Morrison, Prime Minister of Australia, 'Making suicide prevention a national priority', (media release, 8 July 2019), https://www.pm.gov.au/media/making-suicide-prevention-national-priority

8 WHO, 'Addictive behaviours: Gaming disorder', 14 September 2018, https://www.who.int/news-room/q-a-detail/addictive-behaviours-gaming-disorder#

9 Wada, K., 2022, 'Medicalization of Grief: Its Developments and Paradoxes' in Lester, J.N., and O'Reilly, M. (eds) *The Palgrave Encyclopedia of Critical Perspectives on Mental Health*, Palgrave Macmillan, Cham. https://doi.org/10.1007/978-3-030-12852-4_36-1

10 ABS, *National Survey of Mental Health and Wellbeing: Summary of Results*, 66–71

11 Marano, H., 'Anxiety and Depression Together', *Psychology Today*, 1 October 2003 https://www.psychologytoday.com/au/articles/200310/anxiety-and-depression-together

12   Anxiety and Depression Association of America, 'Medication Options', https://adaa.org/find-help/treatment-help/medication-options; Australian Commission on Safety and Quality in Healthcare , 'Atlas 2015 – 4. Interventions for mental health and psychotropic medicines', 2015, https://www.safetyandquality.gov.au/our-work/healthcare-variation/atlas-2015/atlas-2015-4-interventions-mental-health-and-psychotropic-medicines

13   Horwitz, 'How an age of anxiety became an age of depression'

14   Thangadurai, P., and Jacob, K.S., 2014, 'Medicalizing distress, ignoring public health strategies' in *Indian Journal of Psychological Medicine* 36, no. 4: 351–4, doi: 10.4103/0253-7176.140698, 1; Jaman, P. and Staglin, G.K., 'It's time to end the stigma around mental health in the workplace', World Economic Forum, 9 May 2019, https://www.weforum.org/agenda/2019/05/its-time-to-end-the-stigma-around-mental-health-in-the-workplace

15   Tang, S., Reily, N.M., Arena, A.F., et al., 2022, 'People Who Die by Suicide without Receiving Mental Health Services: A Systematic Review' in *Frontiers in Public Health* 9. https://doi.org/10.3389/fpubh.2021.736948

16   Arvidsdotter, T., et al., 2015, 'Understanding persons with psychological distress in primary health care' in *Scandinavian Journal of Caring Sciences* 30, no. 4: 687–694, doi: 10.1111/scs.12289

17   Pūras, *Report of the Special Rapporteur on the right of everyone to the enjoyment of the highest attainable standard of physical and mental health*, 3: Point 10; 10: Point 49

18   Ashfield, J., 'The Madness of Our Mental Health System' in *Mad In America*, 2019, https://www.madinamerica.com/2018/12/madness-mental-health-system

19   Australia Government, Mental health in Australia: a quick guide https://www.aph.gov.au/About_Parliament/Parliamentary_Departments/Parliamentary_Library/pubs/rp/rp1819/Quick_Guides/MentalHealth accessed 6 Jan 2023

20   Angermeyer, M., and Matschinger, H., 2003, 'The stigma of mental illness: effects of labelling on public attitudes towards people with mental disorder' in *Acta Psychiatrica Scandinavica* 108, no. 4: 304–309, doi: 10.1034/j.1600-0447.2003.00150.x; Corrigan, P., 2004, 'How stigma interferes with mental health care' in *American Psychologist* 59, no. 7: 614–625, doi: 10.1037/0003-066x.59.7.614; Timimi, 'No More Psychiatric Labels'

21   Ashfield, et al., A *Situational Approach' to Mental Health Literacy in Australia*, 8–9

Chapter 9 – Proposing new language

1   Arvidsdotter, et al., 'Understanding persons with psychological distress in primary health care'

2   Ashfield, Macdonald and Smith, A *'Situational Approach' to Suicide Prevention*

3   Ashfield, et al., A *'Situational Approach' to Mental Health Literacy in Australia*, 18

4   Fava, G.A., and Sonino, N., 2017, 'From the Lesson of George Engel to Current Knowledge: The Biopsychosocial Model 40 Years Later' in *Psychotherapy and Psychosomatics* 86, no. 5: 257–259, doi: 10.1159/00047880

5   Ashfield, et al., A *'Situational Approach' to Mental Health Literacy in Australia*; Ashfield, Macdonald and Smith, A *'Situational Approach' to Suicide Prevention*

6   University of Rochester Medical Centre, *The Biopsychosocial Approach*, accessed 7 August 2020, https://www.urmc.rochester.edu/medialibraries/urmcmedia/education/md/documents/biopsychosocial-model-approach.pdf

7   Ashfield, Macdonald and Smith, A *'Situational Approach' to Suicide Prevention*

8   Ashfield, J., et al., A *'Situational Approach' to Mental Health Literacy in Australia*, 14

9   ibid.

10   Smith, P.K., et al., 2008, 'Lacking power impairs executive functions' in *Psychological Science* 19, no. 5: 441–447

11 Randall, M., 2011, 'The Physiology of Stress: Cortisol and the Hypothalamic-Pituitary-Adrenal Axis' in *Dartmouth Undergraduate Journal of Science*, retrieved 26 August 2017; Fink, G., 2016, *Stress: Concepts, Cognition, Emotion, and Behavior: Handbook of Stress. Volume 1*, Cambridge: Academic Press

12 Hockey, M., Rocks, T., Ruusunen, A., et al., 2022, 'Psychological distress as a risk factor for all-cause, chronic disease and suicide-specific mortality: a prospective analysis using data from the National Health Interview Survey' in *Social Psychiatry and Psychiatric Epidemiology*, 57(3) pp. 541–552.
Conclusion: D symptoms, of all levels, were associated with an increased risk of all-cause and CVD-specific mortality while higher PD only was associated with suicide. These findings emphasise the need for lifestyle interventions targeted towards improving physical health disparities among those with PD.
Ashfield, J., Macdonald, J. and Smith, A., 2021, *A 'Situational Approach' to Suicide Prevention: Why we need a paradigm shift for effective suicide prevention*

13 Bellack, A.S., 2005, 'Scientific and Consumer Models of Recovery in Schizophrenia: Concordance, Contrasts, and Implications' in *Schizophrenia Bulletin* 32, no. 3: 432–442, doi: 10.1093/schbul/sbj044; Sklar, M., 2013, 'Instruments for measuring mental health recovery: A systematic review' in *Clinical Psychology Review* 33, no. 8: 1082–1095; World Health Organization, 'Suicide: Key Facts', accessed October 2019, https://www.who.int/news-room/fact-sheets/detail/suicide

14 WHO, *mhGAP Intervention Guide for mental, neurological and substance use disorders in non-specialized health settings (Version 2.0)* Italy, World Health Organization; 2016, https://www.who.int/publications/i/item/9789241549790

15 Harrison, J. and Henley, G., *Suicide and hospitalised self-harm in Australia: trends and analysis*, Canberra: AIHW; 2014, https://www.aihw.gov.au/reports/australias-health/suicide-and-intentional-self-harm; Hawton, K., Rodham, K., Evans, E., et al., 2002, 'Deliberate self harm in adolescents: self report survey in schools in England' in *BMJ* 325: 1207–1211, Mental Health Foundation, 'The Truth about Self-Harm', accessed 24 October 2019, https://www.mentalhealth.org.uk/explore-mental-health/publications/truth-about-self-harm

16 Laye-Gindhu, A., and Schonert-Reichl, K.A., 2005, 'Nonsuicidal Self-Harm Among Community Adolescents: Understanding the "Whats" and "Whys" of Self-Harm' in *Journal of Youth and Adolescence* 34, no. 5: 447–457; Klonsky, D.E., 2007, 'The functions of deliberate self-injury: A review of the evidence' in *Clinical Psychological Review* 27, no. 2: 226–239; Muehlenkamp, J.J., 2005, 'Self-Injurious Behavior as a Separate Clinical Syndrome' in *American Journal of Orthopsychiatry* 75, no. 2: 324–333

17 AIHW, Suicide & self-harm monitoring, https://www.aihw.gov.au/suicide-self-harm-monitoring/data/deaths-by-suicide-in-australia/prevalence-estimates-of-suicidal-behaviours Hawton, K., Bale, L., Brand, F., et al, 2020, 'Mortality in children and adolescents following presentation to hospital after non-fatal self-harm in the Multicentre Study of Self-harm: a prospective observational cohort study' in *Lancet Child Adolesc Health*, Feb 2020;4(2):111–120

18 Isometsä, E.T., & Lönnqvist, J.K., 1998, 'Suicide attempts preceding completed suicide' in *British Journal of Psychiatry*, 173, 531–535

19 Bostwick, J.M., Pabbati, C., Geske, J.R., et al., 2016, 'Suicide attempt as a risk factor for completed suicide: Even more lethal than we knew' in *American Journal of Psychiatry*, 173(11), 1094–1100

20 Beautrais, A. 'Suicides and serious suicide attempts: two populations or one?' in *Psychological Medicine* 31, no. 5 (2001):837; Nock, M.K., et al., 2008, 'Suicide and suicidal behavior' in *Epidemiologic Reviews* 30: 144

21 Raven, M., Smith, A. and Jureidini, J., 2017, 'Suicide and Self-Harm in Australia: Conceptual Map', paper presented at the Royal Australian and New Zealand College of Psychiatrists Congress, Adelaide, May 2017

Notes

22 Uh, S., Dalmaijer, E.S., Siugzdaitet, R., et al., 2021, 'Two Pathways to Self-Harm in Adolescence' in *J Am Acad Child Adolesc Psychiatry*, Dec; 60(12):1491–1500. Witt, K., Milner, A., Spittal, et al., 2018, 'Population attributable risk of factors associated with the repetition of self-harm behaviour in young people presenting to clinical services: a systematic review and meta-analysis' in *Eur. Child Adolesc. Psychiatry* 28, 5–18; Plener, P.L., Schumacher, T.S., Munz, L.M., et al., 2015, 'The longitudinal course of non-suicidal self-injury and deliberate self-harm: a systematic review of the literature' in *Borderline Personal. Disord. Emot. Regul.* 2:2; Hawton, K., Saunders, K.E.A. and O'Connor, R.C., 2012, 'Self-harm and suicide in adolescents' in *Lancet*, 379(9834), pp. 2373–2382

23 McPhedran, S. and De Leo, D., 2013, 'Miseries suffered, unvoiced, unknown? Communication of suicidal intent by men in "rural" Queensland, Australia', *Suicide and Life-Threatening Behavior*: 5; Foster, T., 2011, 'Adverse Life Events Proximal to Adult Suicide: A Synthesis of Findings from Psychological Autopsy Studies' in *Archives of Suicide Research* 15, no. 1: 1–15

24 'Table 1: Intentional Self-Harm Fatalities in Australia by Employment Status and Age Range' in Eva Saar and Thomas Burgess, 'Intentional Self-Harm Fatalities in Australia 2001–2013, Data Report DR16 – 16 (2016) National Coronial Information System', http://malesuicidepreventionaustralia.com.au/wp-content/uploads/2017/01/NCIS-Report-2016_FINAL.pdf

25 McPhedran, S. and De Leo, D., 2013, 'Miseries suffered, unvoiced, unknown? Communication of suicidal intent by men in "rural" Queensland, Australia'

26 Seidler, Z., 'We tell men to open up more. But are we ready to listen?', *Age*, 18 October 2019

27 Public Health Association of Australia, 'Suicide Prevention Policy Position Statement', 2018, https://www.phaa.net.au/documents/item/2819

28 AIHW, '7.3 Suicide prevention activities' in Australian Institute of Health and Welfare, *Australia's Health 2018* (Canberra: AIHW, 2008), https://www.aihw.gov.au/getmedia/1ae10a4a-fa4b-4c22-b9d6-2065e1652ed7/aihw-aus-221-chapter-7-3.pdf.aspx%20Accessed%2024%20Oct%202019

29 Baum, et al., 2022, 'Creating Political Will for Action on Health Equity: Practical Lessons for Public Health Policy Actors' in *Int J Health Policy Manag*, 2022, 11(7) (2020), 947–960; Krakouer & Georgatos, 2020, 'The voice of suicide: a cycle of poverty and government inaction' in *National Indigenous Times*, https://nit.com.au/26-03-2020/1051/the-voice-of-suicide-a-cycle-of-poverty-and-government-inaction; American Public Health Association, 'The Role of Public Health in Ensuring Healthy Communities', 2014, accessed 24 October 2019; Delaware Health and Social Services, 'Prevention Definitions and Strategies', accessed 24 October 2019, https://dhss.delaware.gov/dhss/dsamh/files/pds.pdf

30 Lewis, et al., 'Strategies for preventing suicide'

31 AIHW, Suicide & self-harm monitoring, https://www.aihw.gov.au/suicide-self-harm-monitoring/data/technical-notes/methods

32 Raven, M., Smith, A. and Jureidini, J., 2017, 'Suicide and Self-Harm in Australia: Conceptual Map'

33 ABS, *Causes of Death, Australia*; Public Health Information Development Unit (PHIDU), 'Social Health Atlases: Maps', Adelaide: Torrens University Australia, https://phidu.torrens.edu.au/social-health-atlases/maps

34 ibid.

35 Public Health Information Development Unit (PHIDU), 'Notes on the data: Avoidable mortality by selected cause – 0 to 74 years', Adelaide: Torrens University Australia, https://phidu.torrens.edu.au/component/search/?searchword=Notes%20on%20the%20data:%20Avoidable%20mortality%20by%20selected%20cause%20%E2%80%93%200%20to%2074%20years&searchphrase=all&Itemid=1

36   Nock, et al., 'Suicide and suicidal behavior', 144; Beautrais, 'Suicides and serious suicide attempts: two populations or one?'; Raven, Smith and Jureidini, 'Suicide and Self-Harm in Australia: Conceptual Map'
37   Owens, Horrocks and House, 'Fatal and non-fatal repetition of self-harm', 193; Suominen, et al., 'Completed suicide after a suicide attempt', 563
38   Isometsa and Lonnqvist, 'Suicide attempts preceding completed suicide' in *British Journal of Psychiatry*, 173 1998: 531

Chapter 10 – What we need for more effective suicide prevention in Australia

1   Pūras, D., *Special Rapporteur on the right of everyone to the enjoyment of the highest attainable standard of physical and mental health*, 'Depression: Let's talk about how we address mental health', World Health Day, 7 April 2017 https://www.ohchr.org/EN/NewsEvents/Pages/DisplayNews.aspx?NewsID=21480&LangID=E
2   Macdonald, J. et al., *Can Australia's suicide rates be lowered? A Situational Approach to Suicide Prevention: 2018 Symposium Report*, Men's Health Information and Resource Centre, Western Sydney University http://malesuicidepreventionaustralia.com.au/wp-content/uploads/2018/09/SITUATIONAL-APPROACH-TO-SUICIDE-PREVENTION-SYMPOSIUM-FORMAL-REPORT-Sept-12.pdf
3   Doggett, 'The personal and the political: Why do we find it so hard to direct mental health spending to the people who most need it?'; Stark and Fyfe, 'What lies beyond?'; Barbour, 'Criticism for mental health road show'; Middleton, 'Lobbyists dominate mental health sector'; 'Casino, depression not in conflict: Kennett', *SBS News*; Razer, 'Razer's Class Warfare: reducing depression's "stigma" is cheap, stupid policy'; Smith, A., 2020, 'Situational Approach to Suicide Prevention Monthly Bulletin – Issue 14', (ed. Shravankumar Guntuku), Western Sydney University http://www.mengage.org.au/suicide/situational-approach-to-suicide-prevention-mhirc-issue-14
4   Australian Government Productivity Commission, *Mental Health, Draft Report*, Canberra: Productivity Commission, 2019, https://www.pc.gov.au/inquiries/completed/mental-health/draft 82
5   Ashfield, J. and Smith, A., *The Situational Approach to Suicide Prevention and Mental Health Literacy: Advocating for a new multi-sector and multidisciplinary approach*
6   ibid.
7   NHS, 'Safe Haven Cafe in Aldershot, https://www.england.nhs.uk/mental-health/case-studies/aldershot/; *'The Safe Haven' Aldershot: Evaluation Report*, February 2015, https://www.dorsetccg.nhs.uk/wp-content/uploads/2018/07/Annex-9-Aldershot-safe-haven-evaluation-report.pdf
8   'The Shed', Western Sydney University; John Macdonald, 'MHIRC: The Shed in Mount Druitt', Men's Health Information and Resource Centre, Western Sydney University, http://mengage.org.au/men-s-sheds-research/mhirc-the-shed-in-mount-druitt; Bridie Jabour, 'The Shed: "I keep coming because there are people who listen"', in *Guardian*, 22 February 2017, https://www.theguardian.com/australia-news/2017/feb/22/the-shed-i-keep-coming-because-there-are-people-who-listen
9   Jabour, B., 'The Shed: "I keep coming because there are people who listen"' in *Guardian*, 22 February 2017 https://www.theguardian.com/australia-news/2017/feb/22/the-shed-i-keep-coming-because-there-are-people-who-listen
10 Western Sydney University Success of 'The Shed' leads to 2017 Aboriginal Justice Award 2017 https://www.westernsydney.edu.au/newscentre/news_centre/awards_and_appointments/success_of_the_shed_leads_to_2017_aboriginal_justice_award
11 Western Sydney University, 'The Shed In Mt Druitt: Addressing The Social Determinants Of Male Health And Illness', 2012, https://www.westernsydney.edu.au/__data/assets/pdf_file/0003/1308234/MHIC0437_TheShedMtDruitt_FA_LR.pdf
12 Western Sydney University https://www.facebook.com/centremalehealthwsu/videos/722135291662319/ accessed 4 Jan 2023

Notes

13 Casey, S. and Lewis, A., *Redesigning Employment Services after Covid-19,* Per Capita, 27 April 2020, https://percapita.org.au/our_work/redesigning-employment-services-after-covid-19

14 Ashfield, J., Macdonald, J. and Smith, A., 2017, *Creating a National Data Matrix – For Effective Suicide Prevention,* Australian Institute of Male Health and Studies, http://malesuicidepreventionaustralia.com.au/wp-content/uploads/2017/04/National-Data-Matrix-table_web.pdf

Appendices

1 Ashfield, J., Macdonald, J., Francis, A. and Smith, A., 2017, *A 'Situational Approach' to Mental Health Literacy in Australia: Redefining mental health literacy to empower communities for preventative mental health*, Australian Institute of Male Health and Studies, https://doi.org/10.25155/2017/150517

2 Smith, P.K., Jostmann, N.B., Galinsky, A.D., et al., 2008, 'Lacking power impairs executive functions' in *Psychological Science* 19, no. 5: 441–447

3 Randall, M., 2011, 'The Physiology of Stress: Cortisol and the Hypothalamic-Pituitary-Adrenal Axis' in *Dartmouth Undergraduate Journal of Science*, retrieved 26 August 2017; George Fink, 2016, *Stress: Concepts, Cognition, Emotion, and Behavior: Handbook of Stress Volume 1*, Cambridge: Academic Press

4 Ashfield, J., Macdonald, J. and Smith, A., 2017, *A 'Situational Approach' to Suicide Prevention: Why we need a paradigm shift for effective suicide prevention*, Australian Institute of Male Health and Studies; Hockey, M., et al., 2022, 'Psychological distress as a risk factor for all-cause, chronic disease and suicide-specific mortality: a prospective analysis using data from the National Health Interview Survey' in *Social Psychiatry and Psychiatric Epidemiology*, 57(3) pp. 541–552

Conclusion: D symptoms, of all levels, were associated with an increased risk of all-cause and CVD-specific mortality while higher PD only was associated with suicide. These findings emphasise the need for lifestyle interventions targeted towards improving physical health disparities among those with PD.

5 Bellack, A.S., 2005, 'Scientific and Consumer Models of Recovery in Schizophrenia: Concordance, Contrasts, and Implications' in *Schizophrenia Bulletin* 32, no. 3: 432–442, doi: 10.1093/schbul/sbj044; Sklar, M., 2013, 'Instruments for measuring mental health recovery: A systematic review' in *Clinical Psychology Review* 33, no. 8: 1082–1095; World Health Organization, 'Suicide: Key Facts', accessed October 2019, https://www.who.int/news-room/fact-sheets/detail/suicide

6 WHO, *mhGAP Intervention Guide for mental, neurological and substance use disorders in non-specialized health settings, Version 2.0,* Italy, WHO; 2016, https://www.who.int/publications/i/item/9789241549790

7 AIHW Suicide & self-harm monitoring https://www.aihw.gov.au/suicide-self-harm-monitoring/data/deaths-by- suicide-in-australia/prevalence-estimates-of-suicidal-behaviours

8 Turecki, G., and Brent, D.A., 2015, 'Suicide and suicidal behaviour' in *Lancet* 387, no. 10024: 1227–1239

9 Australian Government Department of Health, 'Suicidality', May 2009, https://www1.health.gov.au/internet/publications/publishing.nsf/Content/mental-pubs-m-mhaust2-toc~mental-pubs-m-mhaust2-hig~mental-pubs-m-mhaust2-hig-sui

10 Balhara, Y.P.S., Verma, R. and Gupta, C.S., 2012, 'Gender differences in stress response: Role of developmental and biological determinants' in *Industrial Psychiatry Journal*, 20(1), p. 4; Ashfield, J., 2010, *Doing psychotherapy with men: Practising ethical psychotherapy and counselling with men*, St Peters, South Australia: Australian Institute of Male Health and Studies

11 Harrison, J. and Henley, G., 2014, *Suicide and hospitalised self-harm in Australia: trends and analysis,* Canberra: AIHW, https://www.aihw.gov.au/reports/australias-health/suicide-and-intentional-self-harm; Hawton, K., Rodham, K., Evans, E., et

193

al., 'Deliberate self harm in adolescents: self report survey in schools in England' in *BMJ* 325, 2002: 1207–1211; Mental Health Foundation, 'The Truth about Self-Harm', accessed 24 October 2019, https://www.mentalhealth.org.uk/publications/truth-about-self-harm

12   Laye-Gindhu, A., and Schonert-Reichl, K.A., 2005, 'Nonsuicidal Self-Harm Among Community Adolescents: Understanding the "Whats" and "Whys" of Self-Harm' in *Journal of Youth and Adolescence* 34, no. 5: 447–457; Klonsky, E.D., 2007, 'The functions of deliberate self-injury: A review of the evidence' in *Clinical Psychological Review* 27, no. 2: 226–239; Muehlenkamp, J.J., 2005, 'Self-Injurious Behavior as a Separate Clinical Syndrome' in *American Journal of Orthopsychiatry* 75, no. 2: 324–333

13   AIHW Suicide & self-harm monitoring, https://www.aihw.gov.au/suicide-self-harm-monitoring/data/deaths-by-suicide-in-australia/prevalence-estimates-of-suicidal-behaviours; Hawton, K., Bale L., Brand F., et al., 2020, 'Mortality in children and adolescents following presentation to hospital after non-fatal self-harm in the Multicentre Study of Self-harm: a prospective observational cohort study' in *Lancet Child Adolesc Health*;4(2):111–120

14   Isometsä, E.T., & Lönnqvist, J.K., 1998, 'Suicide attempts preceding completed suicide' in *British Journal of Psychiatry, 173,* 531–535

15   Bostwick, J.M., et al., 2016, 'Suicide attempt as a risk factor for completed suicide: Even more lethal than we knew' in *American Journal of Psychiatry, 173*(11), 1094–1100

16   Beautrais, A., 2001, 'Suicides and serious suicide attempts: two populations or one?' in *Psychological Medicine* 31, no. 5:837; Nock, M.K., et al., 2008, 'Suicide and suicidal behavior' in *Epidemiologic Reviews* 30: 144

17   Raven, M., Smith, A., and Jureidini, J., 2017, 'Suicide and Self-Harm in Australia: Conceptual Map', Paper presented at the Royal Australian and New Zealand College of Psychiatrists Congress, Adelaide, South Australia, 30 April–4 May 2017

18   Uh, S., et al., 2021, 'Two Pathways to Self-Harm in Adolescence' in *J Am Acad Child Adolesc Psychiatry*; 60(12):1491–1500; Witt, K., Milner, A., Spittal, M.J., et al., 2018, 'Population attributable risk of factors associated with the repetition of self-harm behaviour in young people presenting to clinical services: a systematic review and meta-analysis' in *Eur. Child Adolesc. Psychiatry* 28, 5–18; Plener, P.L., Schumacher, T.S., Munz, L.M., et al., 2015, 'The longitudinal course of non-suicidal self-injury and deliberate self-harm: a systematic review of the literature' in *Borderline Personal Disord. Emot. Regu.*, 2:2; Hawton, K., Saunders, K.E.A. and O'Connor, R.C., 2012, 'Self-harm and suicide in adolescents' in *Lancet*, 379(9834), pp. 2373–2382

19   McPhedran, S. and De Leo, D., 2013, 'Miseries suffered, unvoiced, unknown? Communication of suicidal intent by men in "rural" Queensland, Australia', *Suicide and Life-Threatening Behavior:* 5; Foster, T., 2011, 'Adverse Life Events Proximal to Adult Suicide: A Synthesis of Findings from Psychological Autopsy Studies' in *Archives of Suicide Research* 15, no. 1: 1–15

20   'Table 1: Intentional Self-Harm Fatalities in Australia by Employment Status and Age Range' in Eva Saar and Thomas Burgess, 'Intentional Self-Harm Fatalities in Australia 2001–2013, Data Report DR16 – 16 (2016) National Coronial Information System', http://malesuicidepreventionaustralia.com.au/wp-content/uploads/2017/01/NCIS-Report-2016_FINAL.pdf

21   McPhedran, S. and De Leo, D., 2013, 'Miseries suffered, unvoiced, unknown? Communication of suicidal intent by men in "rural" Queensland, Australia'

22   Seidler, Z., 'We tell men to open up more. But are we ready to listen?', in *Age*, 18 October 2019

23   Public Health Association of Australia, 'Suicide Prevention Policy Position Statement', 2018, https://www.phaa.net.au/documents/item/2819

24   Suicide Prevention Resource Center, 'Topics and terms', accessed 24 October 2019

25   Seidler, Z., 'We tell men to open up more. But are we ready to listen?' in *Age*, 18 October 2019

26 Hawton, K., 'Restricting access to methods of suicide: Rationale and evaluation of this approach to suicide prevention'; Yip, P.S., Caine, E., Yousuf, S., et al., 2012, 'Means restriction for suicide prevention' in Lancet, 379(9834):2393–9

27 Gask, L., 2018, 'In defence of the biopsychosocial model' in *Lancet Psychiatry* 5, no. 7: 548; Papadimitriou, G.N., 2017, 'The "Biopsychosocial Model": 40 years of application in Psychiatry' in *Psychiatriki* 28, no. 2: 107–110; Thorpe, R.J., and Halkitis, P.N., 2016, 'Biopsychosocial Determinants of the Health of Boys and Men Across the Lifespan' in *Behav Med.*; 42(3):129–31. doi: 10.1080/08964289.2016.1191231; McInerney, S.J., 2002, 'What is a good doctor and how can we make one?' in *BMJ* 324 :Deacon, B., 2013, 'The biomedical model of mental disorder: A critical analysis of its validity, utility, and effects on psychotherapy research' in *Clinical psychology review*, 33. 10.1016/j.cpr.2012.09.007

28 Foster, 'Adverse Life Events Proximal to Adult Suicide'

29 Almasi, K., Belso, N., Kapur, N., et al., 2009, 'Risk factors for suicide in Hungary: a case-control study' in *BMC Psychiatry* 9, no. 1; Duberstein, P., Conwell, Y., Conner, K.R., et al., 2004, 'Poor social integration and suicide: fact or artifact? A case-control study' in *Psychological Medicine* 34, no. 7: 1331–1337; Diego De Leo, et al., (eds), 2004, *Suicidal behaviour: Theories and research findings*, Ashland, Ohio: Hogrefe & Huber Publishers

30 Macdonald, J., et al., 2016, 'Pathways to despair: a study of male suicide (aged 25–44) in *Public Health Research* 4, no. 2: 62–70

31 Cosgrove, L. et al., 2018, 'Unexamined assumptions and unintended consequences of routine screening for depression' in *Journal of Psychosomatic Research*, 109, pp. 9–11

32 Lewis, G., Hawton, K., Jones, P., et al., 1997, 'Strategies for preventing suicide' in *Br J Psychiatry*; 171:351–4, PMID: 9373424

33 WHO, 'Towards Evidence-based Suicide Prevention Programmes', 2010

34 Baum, F., Townsend, B., Fisher, M., et al., 2022, 'Creating Political Will for Action on Health Equity: Practical Lessons for Public Health Policy Actors' in *Int J Health Policy Manag*, 11(7), 947–960; Krakouer, M. and Georgatos, G., 2020, 'The voice of suicide: a cycle of poverty and government inaction' in *National Indigenous Times*, https://nit.com.au/26-03-2020/1051/the-voice-of-suicide-a-cycle-of-poverty-and-government-inaction; American Public Health Association, *The Role of Public Health in Ensuring Healthy Communities*, 2014, accessed 24 October 2019; Delaware Health and Social Services, *Prevention Definitions and Strategies*, accessed 24 October 2019, https://dhss.delaware.gov/dhss/dsamh/files/pds.pdf

35 Institute of Medicine (US) Committee on Pathophysiology and Prevention of Adolescent and Adult Suicide; Goldsmith, S.K., et al., (eds), 2002, 'Programs for suicide prevention', in *Reducing Suicide: A National Imperative,* Washington DC: National Academies Press; American Public Health Association, *The Role of Public Health in Ensuring Healthy Communities*; Delaware Health and Social Services, *Prevention Definitions and Strategies*

36 Lewis, et al., 1997, 'Strategies for preventing suicide' (which cites Rose 1992)

37 AIHW, Suicide & self-harm monitoring https://www.aihw.gov.au/suicide-self-harm-monitoring/data/technical-notes/methods

38 Raven, M., Smith, A., and Jureidini, J., 'Suicide and Self-Harm in Australia: Conceptual Map'

39 ABS, *Causes of Death, Australia*; Public Health Information Development Unit (PHIDU), 'Social Health Atlases: Maps', Adelaide: Torrens University Australia, https://phidu.torrens.edu.au/social-health-atlases/maps

40 ibid.

41 Public Health Information Development Unit (PHIDU), 'Notes on the data: Avoidable mortality by selected cause – 0 to 74 years', Adelaide: Torrens University Australia, https://phidu.torrens.edu.au/notes-on-the-data/health-status-disability-deaths/avoidable-deaths

42   AIHW, Suicide & self-harm monitoring https://www.aihw.gov.
     au/suicide-self-harm-monitoring/data/populations-age-groups/
     suicide-indigenous-australians

43   Saar, E., and Burgess, T., 2016, 'Intentional Self-Harm Fatalities in Australia 2001–
     2013', Data Report DR16 – 16, National Coronial Information System

44   McPhedran, S., and De Leo. D., 2013, 'Miseries suffered, unvoiced, unknown?
     Communication of suicidal intent by men in "rural" Queensland, Australia'; Saar and
     Burgess, 'Intentional Self-Harm Fatalities in Australia 2001–2013'

45   ABS '2021 Causes of Death' https://www.abs.gov.au/
     statistics/health/causes-death/causes-death- australia/
     latest-release#intentional-self-harm-deaths-suicide-in-australia

46   ABS Causes of Death, 'Australia 2021 Top 10 risk factors by age, proportion of total
     suicides, by age group'

47   Knox, K., 2013, 'Approaching Suicide as a Public Health Issue' in *Annals of Internal
     Medicine* 161, no. 2: 151–152

48   Australian Institute of Male Health and Studies, *Clarification of Some Key Terms and
     Definitions in Suicide Prevention*, 2017, http://aimhs.com.au/cms/uploads/Guidelines_
     DefinitionsJan17v3.pdf

49   Nordt, C. et al., 2015, 'Modeling suicide and unemployment: a longitudinal analysis
     covering 63 countries, 2000–11' in *Lancet Psychiatry* 2, no. 3: 239; Haw, et al.,
     'Economic recession and suicidal behaviour'; Reeves, et al., 'Economic shocks,
     resilience, and male suicides in the Great Recession'

50   Hengartner, M.P., 2017, 'Methodological flaws, conflicts of interest, and scientific
     fallacies: Implications for the evaluation of antidepressants' efficacy and harm' in
     Frontiers in Psychiatry, 8

51   Welsh, H.G., Schwartz, L.M., and Woloshin, S., 2011, *Overdiagnosed: Making People
     Sick in the Pursuit of Health*, Boston: Beacon Press; van Dijk, et al., 'Medicalisation and
     Overdiagnosis'

52   Viola, S. and Moncrieff, J., 2016, 'Claims for sickness and disability benefits owing to
     mental disorders in the UK: Trends from 1995 to 2014' in *BJPsych Open*, 2(1), 18–24

53   SafeWork Australia Mental Health: https://www.safeworkaustralia.gov.au/topic/
     mental-health, accessed 13 May 2020
     Approximately $543 million is paid in workers' compensation for work-related
     mental health conditions

54   Mazza, et al., 'Clinical guideline for the diagnosis and management of work-related
     mental health conditions in general practice'

55   WorkSafe Victoria Mental Injury Support: https://www.worksafe.vic.gov.au/
     mental-injury-support

56   RACGP Work related mental health conditions: https://www.racgp.org.au/clinical-
     resources/clinical-guidelines/guidelines-by-topic/view-all-guidelines-by-topic/
     mental-health/work-related-mental-health-conditions

57   MLC Life Insurance, 'Dealing with depression and anxiety'

58   Australian College Of Applied Professions – Nationally Representative Survey
     Of Australian Workers: https://www.acap.edu.au/wp-content/uploads/2021/12/
     Executive-Summary-ACAP-results-002-1.pdf
     More than half (53%) of Australian workers would hide their mental or physical
     health condition so that they would not be judged or discriminated against. This is
     the equivalent of 6.3 million Australian workers.

59   Acclaimed Workforce data shows 50% of employees are afraid to reveal their mental
     health issue at work, 9 Feb 2022

60   Patty, A., 'Poor understanding of mental health stifles employment', in *SMH*, 16 July
     2021

61   ABS, '6362.0 – Employer Training Expenditure and Practices'

62   MLC Life Insurance, 'Dealing with depression and anxiety'; Workplace Mental Health Institute, 'Mental Health First Aid Australia'

63   Degerman, D., 'Mental health: it's not always good to talk', in *Conversation*, 19 January 2023

64   McPhedran, S., and De Leo, D., 2013, 'Miseries suffered, unvoiced, unknown? Communication of suicidal intent by men in "rural" Queensland, Australia'; Seidler, 'We tell men to open up more. But are we ready to listen?'

65   Chandler, A., 2021, 'Masculinities and suicide: unsettling "talk" as a response to suicide in men', *Critical Public Health*: 1–10

66   ibid.

67   Indigenous Mental Health & Suicide Prevention Clearinghouse, 'Social & emotional wellbeing', Australian Institute of Health and Welfare, 2022, https://www.indigenousmhspc.gov.au/topics/sewb, accessed 5 February 2023

68   Smith, A., 'Focus on individual wellbeing doesn't help', *Guardian*, 8 May 2021, accessed 5 February 2023, https://www.theguardian.com/society/2021/may/08/the-self-help-cult-of-resilience-teaches-australians-nothing

69   Seltzer, L.F., 2010, 'Anxiety and Depression – First Cousins, At Least', Pt 1 of 5 in *Psychology Today*, published 19 May; Harvard Medical School Harvard Health Publishing, 2018, 'Anxiety and physical illness', accessed 25 October 2019; Rice, F., van den Bree, M.B.M., and Thapar, A., 2004, 'A population-based study of anxiety as a precursor for depression in childhood and adolescence' in *BMC Psychiatry* 4, no. 43; Goldberg, D. and Fawcet, J., 2012, 'The importance of anxiety in both major depression and bipolar disorder' in *Depression and Anxiety* 29, no. 6: 471–478; Cole, D.A., Peeke, L.G., Martin, J.M., et al., 1998, 'A longitudinal look at the relation between depression and anxiety in children and adolescents' in *Journal of Consulting and Clinical Psychology* 66, no. 3, 451–460; Watson, D., 2005, 'Rethinking the mood and anxiety disorders: A quantitative hierarchical model for DSM-V' in *Journal of Abnormal Psychology* 114, no. 4: 522–536; Shorter, E., and Tyrer, P., 2003, 'Separation of anxiety and depressive disorders: blind alley in psychopharmacology and classification of disease' in *BMJ* 327: 158–160

Index

Index

Wakefield Press is an independent publishing and
distribution company based in Adelaide, South Australia.
We love good stories and publish beautiful books.
To see our full range of books, please visit our website at
www.wakefieldpress.com.au
where all titles are available for purchase.
To keep up with our latest releases, news and events,
subscribe to our monthly newsletter.

Find us!

Facebook: www.facebook.com/wakefield.press
Twitter: www.twitter.com/wakefieldpress
Instagram: www.instagram.com/wakefieldpress